Obesity

It might not be ALL your fault, but it IS your problem ...

A comprehensive look at obesity--its causes, its historical and cultural evolution, its health risks and alternative approaches to its successful management

by Dorothy S. Mukherjee, RN, BA

Obesity

It Might Not Be **ALL** Your Fault, But It **IS** Your Problem ...

Dorothy S. Mukherjee, RN, BA

Although I'm really fat you see
That's not the way I want to be

They say my mouth is really big
It doesn't mean that I'm a pig

It's veggies all I really eat
And sometimes, maybe...yea, I'll cheat

And 'though I really love to swim
Even that doesn't make me trim

When in the water, very large
Mistaken often for a barge

My friends they say, "There's no dispute ...
...you're fat, **BUT OH SO VERY CUTE.**"

--*Poetry and Art by Dieter Carlton*

INTRODUCTION

As a little girl, I was overweight and awkward. My mother used to tell me how everyone commented about my slowness in learning to walk. She said that I took deliberate and careful steps because my legs were so large that I could not go very fast. I had several brothers and sisters, all of whom, unlike me, developed thin and athletic. One of my sisters became a basketball star and later a basketball coach and my other sister became a high-school dancer and majorette. My youngest brother became a wrestling champ while my other brother played basketball. But me … I was the quintessential "queen of the awkward" and was shunned accordingly. I simply could not compete with my brothers and sisters so they usually left me to myself.

During my grade school and middle school years, I was teased and shunned by my peers, as I was too slow and sluggish to compete in sports or even play competitively with my peers. I had a few friends most of whom were overweight just like me, so I was thankful at least to have a small support group. Although my parents were very supportive of me, I would often agonize when being fitted for clothing—the chubby sizes, of course.

Despite my childhood obesity, I somehow grew up instead of out during my teenage years, probably the result of faster growth hormones. In fact, my weight problem almost disappeared during high school, and I even began to engage actively in sports. Although I still could not compete with my brothers and sisters, I was at least better than average in most sports activities.

I was encouraged by the fact that my weight was healthy for most of my young adult life. Then at age 36 my health took a major turn. It all began after I underwent an emergency hysterectomy operation, the result of which required continual estrogen hormone therapy. This was exacerbated by the fact that I was injured in a car accident that left me incapacitated for six months. Later, I was diagnosed with hypothyroidism, ulcerative colitis and Type II diabetes. These conditions left me weak and poorly motivated, resulting from the medication required to control them. I soon became overweight again. In fact, I eventually gained so much weight that at one point I topped 250 pounds. I was FAT and tried many fad diets and exercise programs to no avail. Feeling doomed to a life of obesity, I eventually underwent bariatric surgery (which I cover in my section in this book on treatments for obesity).

While my life's experience with obesity is unique, in and of itself, it is certainly not uncommon. Today, in fact, it is more common than ever, especially among children and young adults. My own children have struggled with obesity most of their lives and are now among a growing population of young adults that are dealing with this problem. Indeed, although obesity may not be your fault, it's your problem.

Because most of my family members have struggled with obesity at some point in their lives, I became passionately interested in this growing problem, so much in fact, that I began studying its causes and the many approaches to its resolution. I rummaged through hundreds of articles and research studies many of which contradicted each other. I even enrolled into diet fad programs and clinical therapies only to discover that, no matter what you do, if you are predisposed to it, the battle with obesity can be likened to a salmon swimming upstream. This is not necessarily "doomsday" rhetoric. On the contrary, it's simply what it is—if you are fat, most of the time it's just not all your fault. Instead, it's really a combination of factors that include genetic predisposition, metabolism, compelling lifestyle, environment, social convention and many other factors which I will discuss at great length in this book.

This book was purposely arranged to walk the reader through a logical course from the problem to its solution—obesity and how to deal with it, or perhaps how to live with it. The book is divided into three distinct sections. **Section I** is all about obesity and its functional causes and effects. This section describes the clinical condition itself, how it is measured, its causes and its associated risk factors and relationship to other medical conditions. **Section II** gives a discussion on the history of obesity, its mythology and its social and economic development throughout the world. This section is intended of offer a comparative as well as a developmental look at obesity across cultural, social, chronological lines and even religious and philosophical lines. Finally, **Section III** gives a thorough discussion on treatments, protocols and methods of dealing with obesity. This section focuses on the various methods, both personal and professional, that are employed to manage and/or cure obesity.

Order this book online at www.trafford.com
or email orders@trafford.com

Most Trafford titles are also available at major online book retailers.

Printed in the United States of America.

ISBN: 978-1-4269-5529-7 (sc)

Trafford rev. 04/11/2011

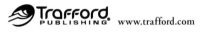 www.trafford.com

North America & international
toll-free: 1 888 232 4444 (USA & Canada)
phone: 250 383 6864 ♦ fax: 812 355 4082

Contents

Section I

The Basics of Obesity

Chapter 1--*Measures of Obesity*

So just what is obesity? Although the answer to this question depends upon a great many things as will be explained later in this book, as a practical matter, obesity is defined quite simply as an excessive amount of body fat. Having said that, anyone with the presence of mind to argue this point can ask us to define what is meant specifically by excess body fat. Indeed, all of us have body fat to a certain extent to insulate us from injury or exposure to the elements. Women have actually more natural body fat than men assuming that both are of normal body mass. In fact, a woman of normal weight stores almost twice the amount of body fat than does a man because this is required for normal ovulation and reproduction.

Most of us can readily see when someone is overweight, especially if that person is very large or, to put it in more colloquial terms, this person is just plain "fat"; but, sometimes one can be overweight and not really be considered "fat". On the other hand, some people can be considered fat or large but are really not overweight. Given these interesting disparities we must somehow address the definition of obesity in scientific terms. If we focus solely upon body fat, the answer as to whether or not someone is truly overweight is not really clear. Recall that woman really have more body fat than men of equal mass. In fact, the average amount of body fat as a percent of body mass for a female is about 27%. By contrast, the body fat content of the average male is about 15% of his total body mass. As we shall learn later in this text, these percentages are actually higher than what would be considered normal body fat in either males or females. Body mass, in this case, refers to the total constitution of one's body; thus, the determination of whether or not a person is obese will depend upon the amount of fat this person carries as a percentage of his/her total body mass. This is also dependent upon a standard or basis on which such a computation should be made, this basis being what we would consider as "normal" body mass.

Before actually exploring the scientific aspects of obesity, it is important to understand a little more about body mass. If we simply use weight as an indicator of obesity, this is not necessarily a precise measure. Fat actually weights less than bone or muscle by volume. It even weighs less than water. By this distinction alone, then a body-builder with a body mass consisting of only 8% fat could easily be regarded as being fat if only weight is employed to measure obesity, in this case. Then too, we must consider also the person's height as well as body frame and bone structure. In fact, it is conceivable that two persons can each be of equal weight and height, yet have vast differences in their distribution of body mass. For example, given a weight of 180 pounds and height of six feet, a sedentary individual will likely even look and be literally defined as obese compared to a well-developed athlete. The point to all of this is that one should not be overly concerned about weight as measured by a common bathroom scale nor should one, on the other hand, dismiss the possibility of having a weight problem if he/she doesn't appear perceptively fat.

A. Definition of Obesity

When we talk about obesity, in most cases, we're referring to someone who is clearly fat or, to put it more gently, somewhat who is, by varying degrees of severity, simply overweight. But being overweight and obese are really two very distinct conditions. Being merely overweight is perhaps embarrassing and something most of us probably deal with from time to time. Obesity, on the other hand, is a serious medical condition and one that must, for the sake of health, be managed and somehow cured. In order to understand obesity, we must have a specific frame of reference from which to best describe this condition.

As a general rule, when we think of obesity we are referring to an overabundance or dangerous accumulation of fat, or put more scientifically—an excessive amount of adipose tissue, in the body. Fat manifests itself in the way we appear, the way we behave and certainly the way we feel. As fat accumulates in our bodies, it eventually begins to take its toll on our daily lives, making us more sluggish and sedentary. These conditions will tend to worsen the accumulation of fat—so, the fatter we become, the fatter still. Fat itself is not especially bad. In fact, our bodies need a certain amount of fat to survive. Fat is especially important for regulating body temperature. Fat also cushions and insulates body tissue and organs and provides a means of temporarily storing energy. A benchmark of fat content by the percentage of total body mass is given by the classifications indicated in **Table I** below.

Table I: Body Fat Percentages to Total Body Mass		
__Classification__	Female	Male
Minimum Essential Fat	10% to 12%	2% to 4%
Athletes	14% to 20%	6% to 13%
Physically Fit	21% to 24%	14% to 17%
Acceptable	25% to 31%	18% to 24%
Overweight	32% to 35%	25% to 29%
Obese	More than 35%	More than 30%

The percentage of body fat in **Table I** refers to the proportion of weight in fat content to the body's total weight. As we proceed further in this chapter, weight will be referred to as body mass. Now, it is important to understand that the percentage benchmarks recorded in **Table I** do not necessarily apply to all persons all of the time. For example, fat content tends to vary, even in normal individuals, by the season of the year and even by geographic region. During the winter months, more fat is needed to help raise body temperature through greater insulation. On the basis of this interesting notion, it is likely that Inuit Eskimos will need more body fat than Polynesian fishermen. Fat density can also vary by race. For example, suppose that a study of several persons of different race classification revealed that they each had the same average amount of fat content. With this in mind, the African-Americans among subjects will have a lower average percentage of body fat to total body mass because their bone density is much greater than that of the average Caucasian. Asians will fall on the other end of this scale. In fact, because of their porous bone density Asians will have a higher average body fat percentage to total body mass than either Caucasians or African-Americans. **Table II** gives a more precise distribution of body fat percentages, based upon this notable distinction.

Table II: Body Fat Percentages by Race						
Class	Males			Females		
	African-American	Caucasian	Asian	African-American	Caucasian	Asian
Minimum	1.6 to 4.7	1.7 to 4.9	2.4 to 5	4.8 to 6.2	8.8 to 12.2	11.3 to 14
Athletes	4.8 to 11.1	5 to 11.6	7.2 to 16.25	6.2 to 10.3	12.3 to 18.4	14.1 to 23.5
Fit	11.2 to 14.3	11.7 to 14.9	16.8 to 21.3	10.4 to 12.4	18.5 to 21.9	23.6 to 28.2
Normal	14.4 to 19.9	15 to 20	21.6 to 30	12.5 to 16	22 to 27.9	28.3 to 36.3
Overweight	20 to 23.2	20.8 to 24.2	30 to 36.25	16 to 18.6	28.1 to 31	36.4 to 41
Obese	More than 23.2	More than 24	More than 36.25	More than 18.6	More than 31	More than 41

Noting the information in Tables I and II, for most of us this should beg the question as to just where each of us falls within the ranges given. Usually, obesity or, for that matter, just being overweight is fairly obvious when we look at ourselves in the mirror, but it's not always obvious when we stand on a scale—that is, unless we know how to use our weight to determine whether or not we are indeed obese or overweight. On the other hand, we might be of normal weight yet consider ourselves obese merely by the perception of how we look. The body can trick us into thinking that we're obese in a number of ways. Abdominal distention resulting from an over-accumulation of digestive gases can significantly impact our appearance. This is true also with the accumulation of fluid. Both of these conditions are usually temporary and may result from injury, metabolic changes occurring in the body or just simply from what we eat and drink.

B. Obesity and Body Mass

The preceding discussion was intended as food for thought (no pun intended) and a way of introducing this business of obesity with an interesting and certainly complex problem—how to accurately measure obesity. We can't just look at someone and assert that this person is obese. It gets even more complicated when you consider the enormous implications of obesity on a person's general health and well-being. Consequently, if we misinterpret someone's body mass, we could easily miss the opportunity to prevent related health issues from complicating this person's condition. Indeed, obesity itself is not the problem. It's how obesity can foster the onset of other, even more serious medical conditions, such as heart disease, stroke, and diabetes.

1. The Quetelet Body Mass Index (BMI)

Although there are many ways in which to measure obesity, some certainly more complex and even more extensive and expensive than others, the most common and widely accepted measure of obesity is known as the **Body Mass Index (BMI)**. The BMI is also known as the **Quetelet Index** or the **Quetelet BMI** after its inventor, Belgian mathematician Lambert Adolpho Quetelet. The BMI is somewhat controversial in that it is a highly generalized indication of body mass; however, it does provide at least a baseline indication of one's degree of obesity. Otherwise, the measure will at least indicate whether or not someone is indeed obese. The formula for measuring body mass by the Quetelet method is summarized

The Quetelet BMI

$$BMI(U.S.) = \frac{W \; x \; 703}{h^2}$$

Where; W = weight in pounds, h= height in inches

$$BMI(Metric) = \frac{W \; x \; 10,000}{h^2}$$

Where; W=weight in kilograms, h=height in centimeters

Example: If you weigh 180 pounds and you are 5 ft, 8 inches tall, your BMI would be as follows:

$$BMI(U.S.) = \frac{180 \; x \; 703}{68^2} = \frac{126,540}{4,624} = 27.37$$

In metric equivalent:

$$BMI(Metric) = \frac{81.82 \; x \; 10,000}{172.72^2} = \frac{818,200}{29,832.2} = 27.43$$

with an example in the text box on the preceding page.

The BMI formula in this example is used for U.S. measures, with the value for weight being in pounds. In order to use the BMI for metric equivalents, the numerator would be one's weight given in kilograms times 10,000 (instead of 703). For those who may be intimidated by the mathematics of obesity, we introduce this measure only for illustration purposes; but, as you will discover, it's really easy to use. Although the example above is given in both U.S. and metric equivalents, for the purposes of this book, the U.S. equivalent will be used.

The BMI, in the textbox example above is about 27.37 (U.S.) and about the same in metric equivalent; but, just what does that mean? Before answering this, we must define another important value. To begin with, normal mass is any BMI index value from 18.5 to 24.9. Now, if we take an individual's BMI and divide this by the upper limit of the normal BMI range, this yields a value known as the *BMI Prime*. BMI Prime is the percentage by which an individual is either over or underweight with a value anywhere from 74% to 100% being normal. Given the preceding example, a BMI of 27.37 would be considered overweight, but not necessarily obese. The BMI prime, in this case, is 27.37 ÷ 24.9 = 1.099 or about 110%. **Table III** below provides a summary of BMI indicators for a typical individual five feet, eleven inches tall. The reason we are using a particular height, in this case, is so that we can show relative corresponding weights for illustration purposes. As a general rule, only the first three columns of the table are relevant for all height values.

Table III: Relative Body Mass Index (BMI) for a person 5 feet 11 Inches tall				
Indications	BMI	BMI Prime	Pounds	Kilograms
Severely Underweight	Less than 16.5	Less than 66%	Less than 118	Less than 53.5
Underweight	From 16.5 to 18.4	From 66% to 73%	From 119 to 131	From 53.6 to 60
Normal	From 18.4 to 24.9	From 74% to 99%	From 132 to 180	From 60.5 to 81
Overweight	From 25 to 30	From 100% to 120%	From 181 to 210	From 81.5 to 97
Obese (Class I)	From 30.1 to 34.9	From 121% to 140%	From 210 to 250	From 97.5 to 113
Obese (Class II)*	From 35 to 40	From 141% to 160%	From 251 to 290	From 113.5 to 130
Obese (Class III)*	More than 40	More than 160%	More than 290	More than 130

*Morbidly obese

Even though a BMI Prime of 110% may seem disconcerting, by U.S. Centers for Disease Control (CDC) standards it only means that you are overweight. Being overweight is not necessarily bad as will become clear later in this book. On the other hand, a BMI prime of more than 120% is clearly considered an indication of obesity and a BMI Prime of more than 150% is considered an indication of morbid obesity. The latter condition is a serious health risk and would require immediate therapeutic or surgical management to resolve. It is important to understand that the BMI is always calibrated on a distribution of ranges. Although these ranges allow for certain deviations in actual body characteristics, they do not always provide an accurate indication for all individuals. Consequently the BMI must be regarded only as a statistical estimate of body mass. Even though this indeed a valid consideration, the CDC considers the BMI an accurate indicator to about 93% if correlated across large population groups. This is especially true if such groups are homogenous--that is, if there are similarities among individuals within the population group in terms of various characteristics as shall be explained as we proceed on this important discussion.

The homogeneity of BMI indications is an important consideration especially when attempting to differentiate obesity indicators between males and females, between adults and children, and certainly, across the various population groups by race or ethnicity, geographic concentration, cultural differences and so on. With this in mind, it would not be logical to compare the BMI of an average adult with that of an average child nor that of an average female with that of an average male. Nevertheless, common sense often prevails in these instances. For example, it is clear that children under the age of 18 have not reached their full growth capacity. Moreover, some children grow faster than others and some at different points in their adolescent lives. So to compare a child's BMI to that of an adult may not be statistically significant. Women on the other hand already have a higher body fat ratio than men. Considering that fat has less weight than any other body component, it would follow that a woman of the same weight and height as that of a typical man will likely have a higher proportional fat ratio, even though the BMI for both would be the same.

2. The NHANES III Model

It is clear from the foregoing discussion that the BMI is really only a benchmark or perhaps a starting point for clinicians to begin the process of evaluating an individual's rate of obesity and corresponding health risks. For this and perhaps the only reason, the BMI is extremely important. There are, of course, other, more rigorous approaches to determining body mass, including one that has become a mainstay of mathematical rigor as it relates to obesity. This approach is referred to as NHANES III Anthropometric Reference Model, derived from the **Third National Health and Nutrition Examination Survey**. Just its name is enough to steer us away from its use in common practice; however, it is reputed as being significantly more accurate because it is not a generalized measure like the BMI. Instead, it uses the mass of one's arms, legs and torso as terms in a more rigorous approach to the computation of total body mass. For illustration purposes and to be fair, it is important to at least offer an introductory discussion of the NHANES III model with a functional example.

The NHANES III approach was actually a survey of individuals of similar comparative mass having different physiological, social and ethnic characteristics. These individuals were evaluated using a complex set of criteria. This method helped to overcome the error associated with the Quetelet BMI's generalized approach to weight and height by the way it eliminates the differences that may result from persons of different body characteristics, such as the obvious difference between males and females. It also differentiates between persons having large bone frames and those with average or below average bone frames. It does so by measuring body mass using the length and diameter of one's upper arm and lower leg as well as the person's sitting height along with several other parameters. It also and especially takes into account a person's age. Age is of course a very important consideration for the measurement of body mass as will be discussed in more detail later in this book. In addition to the physiological predispositions of obesity, the NHHANES III model was careful also to approach this problem with special attention to certain behavioral factors such as smoking. It even sought to differentiate obesity across ethnic and cultural lines.

As a practical tool, the NHANES model is far too rigorous for expedient computation without a pre-programmed calculator. It also requires specific site measurements that cannot easily be self-performed. For this reason, we will address an example by use of **Table IV**. This table provides a summary distribution of NHANES III values as derived from the 1988-1994 study of sampled males and females on which the NHANES III model is based. Using this table and adapting it to the Quetelet methodology introduced earlier, we can approach our original example from a different perspective.

Table IV: Average BMI Distribution (NHANES III survey of 1988-94)						
Age	Males			Females		
	Height	Weight	BMI*	Height	Weight	BMI*
20 to 29	69.13	172.48	25.43	64.05	141.68	23.99
30 to 59	69.41	185.46	27.12	64.09	157.52	27.02
60 + years	68.03	176.44	26.86	62.40	149.38	27.03

Table IV: Average BMI Distribution (NHANES III survey of 1988-94)						
Age	Males			Females		
	Height	Weight	BMI*	Height	Weight	BMI*
All Ages	69.13	180.62	26.63	63.66	152.24	26.47

*kg/m^2

For those interested in viewing the table data using the metric numeric standard, in order to convert pounds to kilograms divide the weight values by 2.2. To convert the height from inches to centimeters, multiply inches by 2.54. For example, the metric equivalent of 175 U.S. pounds is $175 \div 2.2 = 79.55$ kilograms. A 5-foot, 4 inch person in the metric equivalent will be $64 \times 2.54 = 165.1$ centimeters tall.

The BMI values in **Table IV** are actually the average weights and heights given as a value in kilograms per meter squared. For example, the average height in meters for all ages from the values in **Table IV** will be $(69.13 \times 2.54) \div 100 = 1.755902$ meters. Since 180.62 pounds is the equivalent of $180.62 \div 2.2 = 82.1$ kilograms, then the BMI would be $82.1 \div 1.755902^2 = 26.63$ kg/m^2. Having now disclosed the average BMI for the weight and heights derived from the NHAINES III survey, we can now approximate the BMI for various weights and heights using the Quetelet approach. Using males as a benchmark for all ages as given in **Table IV**, we can now derive a new BMI formula by converting the Quetelet constant for a BMI of 26.63. (Note: to distinguish the BMI between males and females, we use the subscripts m and f, respectively).

Derivation of the Quetelet BMI to NHANES III survey results

$$if\ BMI = \frac{W\ x\ C}{i^2}, then$$

Then,

$$C = \frac{BMI\ x\ i^2}{W}$$

And, derived for males from TABLE IV, all ages :

$$C = \frac{26.63\ x\ 69.3^2}{180.62} = \frac{127{,}890.31}{180.62} = 709.71$$

Then,

$$BMI_m = \frac{W\ x\ 709.71}{i^2}$$

For females:

$$BMI_f = \frac{W\ x\ 704.09}{i^2}$$

Armed with this adjustment to the Quetelet BMI, let's suppose that the 5 foot 11 inch, 180-pound person given in our previous example is a 35-year old male. Recall that the original Quetelet BMI for this person was 27.37 which, by the distribution of standards given in **Table III** is considered an overweight condition. This person's BMI after the NHAINES III adjustment would be 27.62.

Although these results are certainly more encouraging than those for males, the adjusted BMI, based on the NHAINES III study is still higher for both males and females. The question raised by these adjustments, of course, is whether or not the NHIANES III study is statistically comparable to the methods used by Quetelet to derive his benchmark equation. After all, there are many indications in modern studies that the rate of obesity may have increased since Quetelet's day. In **Section II** of this book, a look at the historical perspective on obesity will suggest that its prevalence in the population may have actually been about the same throughout the ages.

C. Measuring Body Fat

The preceding discussion on the Quetelet and NHAINES models focused specifically upon total body mass as measured by the BMI. This discussion assumed that the higher the BMI the more inherent body fat would be present. But how can we relate this specifically to the standards introduced in **Table I** and **Table II**. Indeed, we must somehow determine what the BMI means in terms of actual body fat content. To do this, several popular approaches have been adopted from studies of body fat by gender and age. Most notable among these is the Deurenberg-Weststrate-Seidell equations as follows.

Males …

$$F_c = (1.51 \; x \; BMI) - (0.7 \; x \; Age) - 2.2$$

$$F_a = (1.2 \; x \; BMI) + (0.23 \; x \; Age) - 16.2$$

Females …

$$F_c = (1.51 \; x \; BMI) - (0.7 \; x \; Age) + 1.4$$

$$F_a = (1.2 \; x \; BMI) + (0.23 \; x \; Age) - 5.4$$

Where, F_c and F_a are the percentages of fat for children and adults, respectively.

Using this formula, a 55 year old adult male with a Quetelet BMI of 24.4 would have a fat content as a percentage of total body mass as follows:

$$F_a = (1.2 \; x \; 24) + (0.23 \; x \; 55) - 16.2 = 25.73\%$$

If this person had a BMI of 30, his body fat percentage would then be 33.65%, and he would thus be considered overweight.

Readers may surmise, at this point, that normal body fat will actually increase with age. Thus, the normal body fat percentage of a 60-year old may be considered abnormal for a 20-year old. In similar fashion, what may be considered excellent for the average female would be otherwise considered abnormal for the average male. We already know that females must bear higher fat content as a percentage of total body mass than males. It is also true that normal body fat content will increase as we get older. The reason for this is that age tends to wear away the body's natural ability to metabolize nutrients. **Table V** below provides an expanded distribution of body fat percentages by age, gender and severity.

Table V: Distribution of Body Fat Percentages by Gender, Age and Severity									
Females					Males				
Age	Excellent	Good	Fair	Poor	Age	Excellent	Good	Fair	Poor
19 – 24	18.9	22.1	25.0	29.6	19 - 24	10.8	14.9	19.0	23.3
25 -29	18.9	22.0	25.4	29.8	25 -29	12.8	16.5	20.3	24.4
30 – 34	19.7	22.7	26.4	30.5	30 - 34	14.5	18.0	21.5	25.2
35 -39	21.0	24.0	27.7	31.5	35 - 39	16.1	19.4	22.6	26.1
40 – 44	22.6	25.6	29.3	32.8	40 - 44	17.5	20.5	23.6	26.9
45 – 49	24.3	27.3	30.9	34.1	45 - 49	18.6	21.5	24.5	27.6
50 - 54	26.6	29.7	33.1	36.2	50 - 54	19.8	22.7	25.6	28.7
55 - 59	27.4	30.7	34.0	37.3	55 - 59	20.2	23.2	26.2	29.3
60+	27.6	31.0	34.4	38	60+	20.3	23.5	26.7	29.8

D. Other Measures of Obesity

Earlier in this subsection, we introduced the body mass disparity that can result from the fact that fat actually weighs less than other body tissue by volume. The reason for this is that other body tissue contains more water per pound than fat and water weighs more than fat. Because about 27% of the body mass of a typical female consists of fat compared to about 15% for that of a typical male, all other factors held constant, the average female would actually have a lower relative body mass than the average male based on this notable distinction. Why? Let's assume, for the sake of illustration, that fat weights about 70% of all other body components and that the weight of our male is 150 pounds. Since about 15% of the male's body mass consists of fat then we must extrapolate this from his total weight. At 180 pounds, of which 15% is fat, then, (180 x .15 x .7) = 18.9 pounds of fat. Because 70% of the 27% of a female's body weight consists of fat weight then by algebraic manipulation, a female with 18.9 pounds of fat would weigh 100 pounds. To check this, (100 x .27 x .7) = 18.9 pounds of fat.

This notable difference demonstrated above makes it clear that relative weights, if taken by themselves by either the Quetelet or NHAINES III methods, may not always give a true picture of one's rate of obesity. If both the male and the female in the preceding demonstration were of equal height and weight, their BMI's would not be significantly different. It complicates matters even more if can be determined that the male's distribution of fat weight is actually greater than that of the female. This would be a case for even more accurate methods of analysis for the determination of obesity.

1. Hydrostatic Weight Determination

Because of the inherent weaknesses of the popular Quetelet and NHAINES III methods for measuring body mass, many physicians and therapist tend subscribe to the more scientific methods. As we have already introduced in the previous discussion, fat actually weighs less than other body tissue. It also weighs less than water. On the basis of this notion, therefore, it is conceivable that the presence, as well as the degree, of body fat can be measured from the amount by which the mass of a person's body will displace an equivalent amount of water. In scientific terms, this is really an application of Archimedes principle of displacement which basically states as follows: (1).The densities of fat mass and fat-free mass are both constant; (2). Lean tissue is denser than water; (3). Fat tissue is less dense than water; therefore, (4). A person with more body fat will weigh less underwater. This principle gave birth to the **Hydrostatic** or buoyancy method of weight determination.

As a comparative measure of body mass, the hydrostatic method can be a very useful weight determinant. Using the average weight of individuals considered as being of normal body mass, a baseline standard is used as a measure against the actual amount of water that is displaced by the individual being measured. In this case, more water will be displaced by individuals having less fat as a percentage of total body mass. This water displacement is measured on a scale which actually shows the amount in inches or centimeters by which the water rises in a tank.

Although the hydrostatic method of weight determination is considerably more precise than either the Quetelet or NHAINES III approaches, it too bears certain fundamental weaknesses. The most obvious of these is that fat displacement can often be influenced by the volume of air in one's body. This is based on the notion that lung capacity will vary from individual to individual. Gas is also displaced in other areas of the body. Digestive gases can differ widely from one person to the next, especially if there are vast differences in diet intake. In fact, digestive gases can even make persons appear overweight even if they are not.

2. Skinfold Thickness Weight Determination

When we introduced the NHAINES III approach to measuring body fat, we were referring specifically to a division of measurement known as anthropometric analysis. The term anthropometric refers to the use of various parts of the human body to evaluate a person's percentage of body fat. The NHAINES III study focused on the dimensions of a person's arms, legs and waist or torso. Another anthropometric method focuses on the organ that stores most of the body's fat—skin. This method is known as the Skinfold Test whereby the skin is compressed or pinched by calipers along various surface areas of the body to determine subcutaneous (under the skin) fat layer thickness. From the resulting measures, complex equations are used to derive the amount of body fat.

The skinfold test is actually a means of statistically estimating total body fat because it only uses the content of adipose tissue in the skin to measure obesity. There are several other areas of the body wherein fat is stored, including visceral adipose tissue or fat deposits within the abdominal cavity. The statistical method used is a type of inferential induction and assumes therefore that there is a direct correlation between the content of fat in the skin and the total amount of fat in the body. In theory, it's sort of like measuring human population characteristics of millions of persons from the evidence of one or more small samples.

3. Bioelectric Impedance Analysis (BIA)

Bioelectric Impedance Analysis (BIA) is based on a very simple principle of electronics. It is a well known fact that electrical conduction is determined by the properties of matter through which a current travels. We know, for example, that electricity travels much more efficiently through water than through wood or through steel than through led. With this in mind, it was determined that electrical current has significantly less resistance when travelling through free-fat mass or muscle which consists of about 73% water than through fat. The reason for this is that fat is anhydrous, meaning that it is almost totally void of water and thus a poor conductor of electricity. The determination of body fat using BIA is done by attaching small conductors to each foot. A small current is passed which extends up one leg, into the abdomen and back down the other leg while an instrument much like an oscilloscope, measures the amount of electrical resistance. When compared to a chart of standards for what is considered normal conduction, the BIA can determine, to a certain extent, the amount of body fat in the person being tested.

4. Near-Infrared Interactance (NIR)

Near-Infrared Interactance or NIR is a relatively inexpensive means of calculating body fat percentages. With this method, which is non-invasive (non-surgical), a digital, infra-red scanner or fiber-optic probe attached to a computerized spectrophotometer is used to measure fat that may exist around various parts of the body. The probe emits an infrared light which passes through the skin, fat and muscle and then bounces back off the dense tissue of the bone. Using the differences in depth or thickness among these three tissue types, the spectrophotometer can estimate the amount of total body from a sampled area of the body. The site most commonly scanned with this method includes the biceps or upper arm area. When correlated to fat percentage calculations using other methods, the NIR methods has been fairly consistent in measuring body fat; however, its validity is still under scrutiny and study.

5. Dual Energy X-Ray Absorptiometry (DEXA)

Dual-Energy X-Ray Absorptiometry or DEXA is a method of analyzing fat based upon its density in relation to other body tissue, including the bone. DEXA is also sometimes called bone densitometry because it is used primarily to measure bone density and loss. Although DEXA is used to evaluate many other medical conditions, especially those related to the bone, it can also be used to measure the density of other types of body tissue, including fat and then easily differentiated among them to establish their proportions to total body mass. Unlike NIR, DEXA is an expensive procedure because it uses ionizing radiation, X-Ray, to scan the entire body with a scanner much like computer tomography (CT) or magnetic resonance imaging (MRI). A DEXA scan also takes comparatively longer than NIR, but is much more accurate as a measure of fat content.

E. Chapter Summary

As we should now know, obesity is a condition derived from the accumulation of more body fat than the is required for normal human functions. In general, the amount of essential body fat in males should not exceed 15% of total body mass and, among females, 27% of total body mass. Any amount of body fat in excess of these benchmarks determines a range of conditions from mildly overweight to morbidly obese.

In order to determine the degree by which an individual may be overweight several popular measures have been developed. Among these are the Quetelet Body Mass Index (BMI) and the NHANES III Model. Both of these determine the extent by which an individual may be overweight by differentiating one's height and weight against a commonly accepted standard. In addition to overall body mass, there are also several mathematical measures used to determine the actual amount of body fat as a proportion to total body mass.

Although the mathematical models for measuring body fat can be used readily by most individuals, they only provide a rough estimate of body fat content. The more accurate methods for measuring body fat require third-party intervention and management. These are the clinical interventional methods of measuring body fat. Among the popular clinical measures used to determine body fat content are Hydrostatic Weight Determination, Skinfold Thickness, Biometric Impedance Analysis, Non-Infrared Interactance and Dual Energy X-Ray Absorbtiometry.

Key Points:

1. Obesity results from an over-accumulation of fat in the body
2. Body Mass is equal to your weight in pounds x 703 divided by the square of your height in inches
3. The acceptable amount of fat in females is 27% of total body mass and in males 15%
4. The acceptable amount of body fat to total body mass will increase with age

Chapter 2--*The Mechanics of Obesity*

In order to best understand the mechanism of obesity, it is important for us to review how the body works to give us the energy we need to survive. Like anything else that requires movement, some form of fuel is needed to energize this process. Gasoline is used to automate cars, boats, planes and so on just as electricity is used to operate the many things we use in our daily lives. If we want to animate a child's toy or make a flashlight work, we usually need batteries. Well, our bodies are just that, BATTERIES. Strange as that may sound, like the chemical acids in a standard flashlight battery, our bodies too are composed of a complex array of chemicals that generate the electricity we need to survive. But much like any battery, if a way is not provided by which to charge and recharge its stored energy, it will eventually become depleted and the battery will die.

Humans charge their internal batteries by consuming the nutrients needed to survive. These nutrients come in various forms we call food and, of course, water or some type of beverage. When our body needs nourishment, it tells us so in the form of hunger and thirst. When we are full, our body then tells us to stop eating and drinking. In a normal, healthy individual this cycle of survival should keep our bodies in perfect working condition and pretty much at the same weight most of our lives. So then why do we get fat? To answer this question there are a few things we must know about how the body manages what we consume.

A. The Digestive Process

If we go to our garage or driveway and just look at our car, we see a complex mass of steel, rubber, plastic and glass that simply sits there and does nothing. But, we know that it is possible to animate this car. Indeed, we can open the door, sit down in the driver's seat, insert and turn the ignition key and suddenly the car comes to life. We can now move very quickly to where we want to go by the complex operation of various engineered components that give our car motility or motion. Fuel is injected, mixed with oxygen and ignited by an electrical charge to form combustion which moves the pistons that drive the transmission and move the car. Although this is a simplified description of the mechanics of an automobile, it can to some extent be used analogously to describe how our bodies work. Drawing a few parallels, our brain can be viewed as the driver of the car and the food we eat, the gasoline required to put the car into motion. Like the gasoline in a car, the food we eat provides the energy needed by our bodies to operate all of the mechanisms that give us life. The general term used to describe this mechanism--all of the various components of the body and how they work to give us life is called *physiology*.

Wouldn't it be great if our bodies could be like that of a car—always the same size. With a car, you can't overfill the gas tank; but, with the human body, you can—you can take in too much fuel. Instead of the fuel being spilled over and onto the ground, what isn't expelled as human waste is just stored, and it's done so in the form of FAT. Scientist really haven't figured out why the mechanism of getting fuel to give us life can't just be constant like the capacity of a car's fuel tank. It is still not clear why there is not a trigger or physiological mechanism that keeps our body exactly the same mass. Indeed, we understand certainly that our body can tell us when we're hungry and also when we're full. What our body can't tell us whether the kind of fuel we are using is efficient or inefficient. A car can use regular or high octane fuel. This fuel can also be pumped full of additives to make the car run cleaner and more efficiently, but the car still stays the same size and shape. If we consume too much high octane food, that is, food having more calories than our bodies can burn, we're simply going to get fat.

1. The Upper Digestive Processing Plant

Although most of us should understand how we process what we consume, a brief review will prepare us for the more advanced mechanics of how we can become obese. To help in describing the digestive system, the reader may want to refer to **Figure 1** on the succeeding page. In general, the instant we put food in our mouths, even though we try to chew it carefully before we swallow it, a chemical known as *saliva* already begins to break it down. It then passes down the esophagus where the muscles in its wall act like ocean waves to drive the food into the stomach by a process known as *peristalsis*. The food is then passed through the *esophageal sphincter* and into the stomach. The esophageal sphincter is a ring-like muscle which acts much like a one-way check valve used by plumbers to prevent water from moving back to where it came from. In the stomach, a hormone known as *gastrin* produces a powerful hydrochloric acid to break the food down into a pea soup-like substance known as *chymus* or *chyme*.

Now very little more than highly acidic soup, the food (chyme) is then passed across into the *duodenum*. The duodenum, also known as the *anterior intestine* or *proximal intestine*, is where various hormones from the pancreas and liver convert it to a state that can be easily absorbed through the walls of the small intestine. As food is passed into the duodenum, a hormone called *secretin* immediately signals the pancreas to produce digestive juices rich in sodium bicarbonate to reduce the acid contents of the food that accumulated in the stomach. At the same time, a hormone called *bile* from the liver is then squeezed out by the gall bladder in order to break fat down much like dish washing detergent does with grease in a frying pan. After all of this, the food is than passed into the *ileum* and *jejunum* (the small intestines) where it is finally absorbed and passed into the blood stream. Whew! This certainly is a magnificent process, the extent of which, when even the slightest bit deficient, can easily contribute to obesity as we shall learn later in this book.

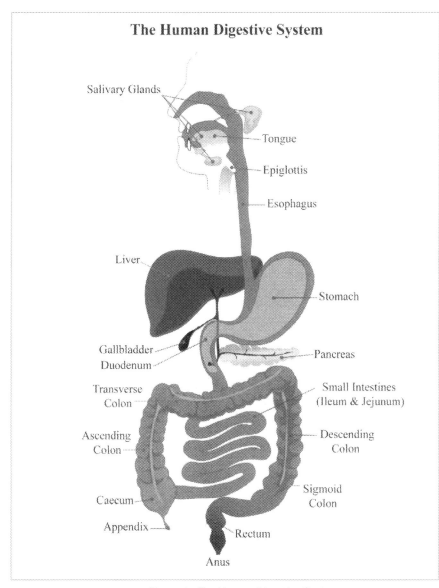

The Human Digestive System

Salivary Glands
Tongue
Epiglottis
Esophagus
Liver
Stomach
Gallbladder
Duodenum
Pancreas
Transverse Colon
Small Intestines (Ileum & Jejunum)
Ascending Colon
Descending Colon
Caecum
Sigmoid Colon
Appendix
Rectum
Anus

Figure 1: The Human Digestive System

2. The Lower Digestive Processing Plant

A large part of what we eat is actually bulk or what is often called "roughage". This inert matter is composed of undigested *polysaccharides* that cannot be further digested and are thus passed through the small intestine and into the large intestine or colon as waste. The colon is a short, but very large organ that begins where the small intestines enter its contents into the *caecum*, up the *ascending colon*, across the *transverse colon* to the *descending colon* and into the *sigmoid colon*. The most common usage of digestive waste is fiber. Even though the colon processes waste, it is interesting to note that it contains hundreds of species of bacteria which actually break some of the waste down and absorb it through its walls and into the blood stream as vitamins. Nevertheless, only a small percentage of the body's vitamin needs are actually generated by this process. These include Vitamin K and biotin which will be discussed in the next subsection on calories. Of course, at the very end of the digestive process is the *anus* or *rectum* through which bulk waste is finally passed. The entire path that food takes from the mouth to this rather unflattering component of the body is a 30-foot passage, including the esophagus, stomach, small intestine and large intestine, known as the *alimentary canal*. In short, the digestive process is quite "alimentary".

B.   All About Calories

When we eat and drink to nourish our bodies, this is done to give us the energy needed to sustain ourselves. The body is capable of extracting all of the necessary nutrients from the food we eat and what we drink and then expels the rest as waste. Our digestive system efficiently filters and converts what we eat and drink to energy in the form of heat. Some of the foods we eat actually burn hotter or faster than others and thus take less time to digest. For example, it takes the body much longer to burn a chocolate cake than it does to burn an apple, even though both may be of similar mass. This is sort of like the difference between high octane and regular unleaded fuel for a car. Both are still the same quantity, but high octane fuel, which costs more, should make the car run more efficiently. If we think of the food we eat as energy in a commonly understood form, the amount of heat energy in a six ounce cheesecake is approximately enough to burn a 60-Watt light bulb for about one and a half hours. A McDonald's "Big Mac" provides enough energy to drive a compact car nearly 90 miles.

These astonishing revelations are not mythological to be sure. They were calculated using a common measure of energy known as the *Calorie*. A calorie is actually a unit of energy or, put in more relevant terms, a unit of heat much like Fahrenheit or Celsius when they are used to measure temperature. A calorie by definition is actually the amount of heat it takes to raise one gram of water, one Celsius or, in the U.S. standard, .0325273 ounces of water 1.8 degrees Fahrenheit. To put this in relative perspective, a U.S. gallon of regular unleaded gasoline contains about 31,000,000 calories. The usage of the term calories has always been a misnomer when applied to the measurement of food. A food calorie is actually a *kilocalorie*. For example, when we talk about something having 300 calories, this is actually 300 kilocalories or 300,000 real calories. For the sake of simplicity and generally accepted or colloquial usage, when the term calorie is used in this book it, of course, is referring to kilocalories.

Another way to express calories or kilocalories is by considering what it takes to boil water. As we should all know, water boils at 212 degrees Fahrenheit (or 100 degrees Celsius) at sea level or, more accurately, at the elevation in which the atmospheric pressure is 29.92 inches of mercury or about 1 atmosphere. The boiling point decreases about 1 degree Celsius for every 285 meters of elevation. Given what we've learned so far about calories, to raise the temperature of one cup (8 ounces of water) to 212 degrees we need to do a little math. We know that one calorie is what it takes to raise the temperature of .032573 ounces of water 1.8 degrees Fahrenheit. So then it would take (8 ÷ .032573 x 1.8) = 442 calories to raise the temperature of one cup just 1.8 degrees Fahrenheit. If we assume that the water temperature is already 33 degrees Fahrenheit (just above the freezing point) then it takes (212 -33) ÷ 1.8 x 442 = 43,954.44 calories or about 43.95 kilocalories to bring 8 ounces of water to a boil.

The entire system of measuring food energy by the use of calories is based on a very simple principle. In general, our bodies need three types of nutrients: fat, carbohydrates and protein. Together, these three nutrients are known as building blocks. If we know how much of these nutrients are contained in a quantity of food or drink, we can determine how much potential energy is available in this quantity. We know that one gram of fat has 9 calories, one gram of either carbohydrates or protein has 4 calories. Since fat has more than twice the caloric content of either carbohydrates or protein, it will take the body much longer to burn fat. So, when we suggested that it takes longer to burn the energy provided by a chocolate cake than by an apple, it's because the chocolate cake contains more fat than an apple. But fat also comes from carbohydrates as we shall see later.

Since we now know how many calories there are in the three common nutrients we can easily calculate the amount calories contained in a typical food item. For example, when we look at the label on, say, a package of pasta, we might see 4 grams of fat, 38 grams of carbohydrate and 7 grams of protein, this is the equivalent of 103 calories. There are of course other components of food that have little or no nutritional value, such as salt, sugar and various spices. It is also important that the nutrients we eat, despite the number calories contained therein, consist of a proper amount of vitamins and minerals both of which, so to some extent can influence the amount of fat that can be stored in our bodies.

Most of us know how a car burns fuel or, for that matter, how electricity can burn a light bulb, but how the body burns food in the form of energy is not as clearly understood. The reason for this is that it is a very complex process known as *metabolism*. The term, metabolism, will play a significant role in this book, especially when it is used to evaluate obesity. Metabolism is actually a complex chemical reaction by which nutrients are processed to produce energy. Although more about metabolism will be discussed later in this chapter, in general, with the process of metabolism enzymes are natural body chemicals that are used to convert the carbohydrates we eat into glucose and other sugars. These same enzymes convert fats to glycerol and fatty acids and protein into amino acids. This is the body's way of breaking food down to a state that can be easily absorbed into the various cells of the body through the blood stream. Together, these converted nutrients then react to the oxygen content of our cells to release the energy we need.

1. Carbohydrates

Although fat and protein are needed in combination with carbohydrates to give us energy, it is the carbohydrates that actually provide us with the fuel necessary to produce energy just like gasoline is used to operate a car. When passed into the body through the intake of food, a hormone called *amylase* combines with saliva in the mouth to begin immediately converting carbohydrates to a simple sugar known as *glucose*. Glucose is also sometimes called *blood sugar* or *dextrose*, two terms that will have more meaning when we get into the discussion in this book on the risks of obesity. The term carbohydrate is actually a chemical combination used to describe the integration of carbon ("carbo") and water ("hydro"). Glucose then reacts with other chemicals in the body to produce a powerful phosphate called *adenosine triphosphate* or ATP, the chemical that, like the chemicals in a flashlight battery, energizes all of the cells in our body.

Glucose is one of several types of simple sugars which together are known as *monosaccharides*. It is important to understand that glucose is very similar to the sugars that we can take into our bodies directly such as fructose and sucrose, except that glucose is converted from the more complex carbohydrates in food. Sucrose is actually known as a disaccharide because it contains two *monosaccharides;* however, it too is broken down into a monosaccharide because the latter is the only carbohydrate that can be absorbed into cells through the intestinal tract and into the blood stream. Although much of this discussion may seem complex and confusing, it provides a foundation for what we need to understand the mechanism of obesity and the many health risk associated with obesity. In fact, the way in which our body manages simple sugars has a significant bearing one of the most serious potential consequences of obesity—diabetes.

Before moving on, it is important to distinguish *simple* from *complex* carbohydrates. Glucose is actually a simple carbohydrate because it is, in and of itself, a monosaccharide and thus can be directly and immediately absorbed into the intestinal tract and then into the bloodstream. Complex carbohydrates, on the other hand, must be broken down, a process that takes considerably longer than with simple carbohydrates, a factor that is of great importance in the discussion of obesity. Complex carbohydrates or "starches", as they are commonly called, are contained in many of the foods we eat such as potatoes, grains like corn, wheat oats and rice, pasta, etc. Starches are actually used by plants to store their own energy. But, no matter how complex, the starch is still broken down to glucose so that our bodies can absorb it for our source of energy.

It is interesting to note that, since glucose is absorbed immediately into the bloodstream for energy then eating sugar or something high in sugar content like soda or candy will give us an immediate source of energy. In fact, it takes about 30 calories per minute to process a piece of rock candy, but only about 2 calories per minute to process a six-ounce bowl of rice. So why is this so important? Well, our bodies can only burn so many calories per unit of time and this, of course will depend upon how much energy we need based upon the activity in which we are engaged. So, if we take in more calories per minute than our bodies can burn, the excess will be stored as fat until we're eventually able to burn it. The problem is that, sometimes we may take in more calories over time than the body can burn and thus wind up accumulating this stored energy in the form of excess body fat. The immediate effect of consuming sugars is considerably more ominous.

As children, our parents would likely avoid feeding us foods high in sugar content, or they may have simply said to us that if we eat too much candy, "it's bad for you." Although our parents may not have understood the physiological mechanism behind their assertion, the foundation of these assertions is worthy of note. You see, simple carbohydrates in the form of sugar require little or no digestion. Consequently, they are rapidly absorbed into and thus raise the sugar levels of the blood stream-- the so called *blood sugars*. As a natural defense mechanism, in order to prevent the sugar levels from rising too high, the *pancreas* secretes larger amounts of a natural hormone known as *insulin*. The pancreas is a large gland situated near the stomach that aids in the digestive process.

Insulin is one of the most important hormones in our bodies and is actually a protein that helps transfer glucose into our cells. Insulin is both a friend and a foe. As a friend it helps to convert glucose to energy and also to glycogen for storage in the liver and muscles. As a foe, insulin converts excess glucose to FAT. High levels of insulin in the body work very slowly but eventually, after about 2 to 3 hours from the consumption of foods high in sugar content, it could cause the blood sugar levels in the body to venture below normal. This results in a temporary condition known as *hypoglycemia.*

In normal individuals, hypoglycemia is actually a very mild, but temporary, form of insulin shock caused by a rise in the body's adrenaline levels. This condition, while not necessarily serious, can make us nervous and irritable and sometimes, even weak and dizzy. For those of us who have ever eaten a candy bar before exercising (clearly a mistake) we may recall becoming hypoglycemic very quickly. The reason for this is that sugar is more quickly converted to energy when we exercise than when we're at rest. Consequently, the insulin that is secreted by the pancreas begins doing its work to lower the sugar levels after they have already been lowered by the body's higher need for energy. The result is more insulin in the body than it needs, so the insulin actually slows us down until the levels are back to normal. Most professional or well-informed athletes understand the mechanism of hypoglycemia and instead of consuming high quantities of sugar before an event will do what trainers refer to as "carbo-loading". Hours before an event, athletes will eat a large quantity of complex carbohydrates because these carbohydrates are processed very slowly and gradually over time; hence, they are stored and gradually burned in the form of heat energy during the event.

A very important consideration with respect to carbohydrates, especially how carbohydrates relate to obesity, is what happens to the body when sugar levels are too high. Remember that any glucose levels above what the body needs for energy are converted by insulin to fat and, well ... that's one of the many ways we can become obese. If the pancreas cannot secrete enough insulin to manage the over-abundance of sugar, this could result in another condition called *hyperglycemia*. Hyperglycemia in normal persons is usually temporary and largely asymptomatic, so we often never know that we had it. But, if you've ever experienced sudden or frequent episodes of hunger or thirst—this is likely the result of mild hyperglycemia. More serious episodes of hyperglycemia can manifest themselves in the form of cardiac stress and coma. Considerably more will be discussed about both hypoglycemia and hyperglycemia in **Chapter 4** when we explore how these can develop into chronic condition known as diabetes.

2. Proteins

While carbohydrates act like fuel to give us the energy we need, this energy must be processed by the cells in our bodies to do this efficiently. Proteins actually maintain and repair the cells of our bodies for this purpose and are thus known as building blocks. Proteins are actually converted through the digestive process to *amino acids*. It is the amino acids which actually provide the mechanism of reproduction, growth and repair of cells. Although the body can create its own amino acids through simple chemical reactions, these are actually known as non-essential amino acids and have nothing to do with digestion. The essential amino acids, those that are the building blocks of our cells, are derived exclusively from the foods we eat. Essential amino acids are very complex and consist of many different types all having different roles in the cellular metabolism process. For the purposes of this discussion, we will refer to these only as a group, amino acids in general, since they all operate in much the same way.

Amino acids are actually derived from the protein contained in many of the foods we eat including, but to a limited extent, vegetables. Most proteins are contained in milk and meat products. Eggs are a very high source of protein. In fact, proteins from milk, eggs and meats are called *complete proteins* because they contain most of the essential amino acids the body needs.

Unlike the complete proteins, vegetables should really be called incomplete proteins because most of them, such as lettuce, cabbage and rice provide considerably less protein per ounce or gram than the complete proteins. For this reason, those who do not eat meat such as vegetarians must be careful to eat a variety of vegetables that include those containing larger amounts of protein, like nuts and soybeans. In short, the body simply cannot survive solely on a carbohydrate diet, nor can the body survive solely on a protein diet. It must have both to survive.

3. Fat

A book about obesity certainly cannot be complete without a serious and thorough discussion of the principal source of obesity—FAT. Fat is that ugly word that many of us wish would just go away along with its namesake, of course. While fat is a term commonly used to describe how we may appear, it is also a substance contained to a great extent in the foods we eat. Fat alone does not necessarily make us fat, but it contributes extensively to the problem. Fat can derive from both animals as well as from vegetables and is divided into two distinct types— *saturated fats* and *unsaturated fats*. Animal fats are always saturated and are easily recognized because they harden at room temperature. Butter, shortening and lard are examples of saturated fats. Although vegetable oils are considered unsaturated fats, some vegetable oils, like olive oil, can actually contain a mixture of both saturated and unsaturated fats. In order to determine if liquid oils contain any saturated fats, simply refrigerate the oil and the saturated fats contained therein will solidify.

As we shall learn in **Chapter 3**, saturated fats are much less healthy than unsaturated fats, but too much of either over many years may cause serious medical problems. Unsaturated fats can be divided into two categories, *polyunsaturated fat* and *monounsaturated fat*. Although both are better for you than the saturated fats, monounsaturated fats are best for the metabolism of blood cholesterol levels since they lower bad cholesterol while actually raising the good cholesterol levels in the bloodstream. Unsaturated fats can actually be harmful by the way they are processed. For example, some vegetable oils are processed by adding hydrogen to them through a process called hydrogenation to produce a dangerous by product known as *trans-fatty acids*.

As we now know, body fat can not only be produced from an overproduction of glucose as derived from carbohydrates in the digestive process, it can come directly from the foods we eat. But, fat is also an essential food product, especially if we do not get enough carbohydrates in our bodies. Fat is essential for several reasons. First of all fat is needed by the skin and muscles for lubrication and heat insulation. When we consume fat directly it is digested by an enzyme called *lipase* which breaks the fat into *glycerol* and *fatty acids*. These act together to produce *triglycerides* which, like the glucose derived from carbohydrates and amino acids from protein, are the only chemicals that can be absorbed into the blood stream. Although triglycerides are essential elements of body metabolism, like glucose, their overproduction is stored in the body as fat. Fat also provides a medium for certain vitamins called fat-soluble vitamins which actually eat the fat to produce *coenzymes*. Coenzymes react with the natural enzymes in the body to aid in digestion and waste disposal. Fat is also used as a building block, like amino acids, but in this case to insulate and protect cells from injury; and, because fat contains twice the amount of calories than either protein or carbohydrates, it is also a powerful source of static energy after it has been stored in the body.

4. Vitamins and Minerals

In addition to carbohydrates, protein and fat, the body also needs vitamins and minerals to survive, although neither is considered a source of food by itself. Vitamins are essential for body metabolism because they are external sources of nutrition that react chemically in the body to form temporary enzymes. The body uses natural enzymes which are secreted by the various glands that make up our anatomy. The pancreas is the gland that processes the foods we eat into a form that can readily be absorbed into the blood stream. But, the pancreas cannot act alone. It needs some friends in the form of vitamins. For this reason vitamins act cooperatively with the enzymes produced naturally in the body to produce their own enzymes which is why they are call coenzymes. Most vitamins are not produced in our bodies, instead we must obtain them from what we eat and drink. In fact, Vitamin D is the only one actually produced by our bodies but not in sufficient quantities to survive.

There are actually two types of vitamins, those that are *water-soluble* and those that are *fat-soluble*. Water soluble vitamins stay in the body until they are expelled via the body's sweat glands or through the kidney and bladder as urine. These vitamins "hang out" so to speak just long enough to release the enzymes and coenzymes needed by the body to aid in metabolism. Because water-soluble vitamins are temporary, we must frequently eat the foods that contain them. Fat soluble-vitamins are those that are actually stored in the fat contained in our bodies and released as we need them. This is one of the reasons why it is important to have at least some fat in the body. You may be thinking at this point that, if we are fat, we should have plenty of vitamins to keep us healthy. Actually, there are only four essential fat-soluble vitamins, Vitamin A (Retenol), Vitamin D (Calciferol), Vitamin E (Tocopherol) and Vitamin K (Menaquinone). The body still needs the water-soluble vitamins, including Vitamin B Complex, Vitamin C (Ascorbic Acid), Pantothetic Acid and Biotin. These vitamins, including those that make up the Vitamin B Complex, are the 13 essential vitamins needed by the body.

This discussion of vitamins is an important consideration in addressing the problem of obesity. The reason for this, as shall be addressed more in detail in Section III of this book, is that often the way obesity is managed is done so through diets which tend to deplete or even omit one or more essential vitamins. This in turn can result in other, often more serious medical conditions than the state of obesity itself. Lack of essential vitamins can cause many diseases. These are noted, along with other information about each of the 13 essential vitamins in **Table VI** below.

Table VI: Essential Vitamins and Their Properties					
#	Vitamin	Sources	Needed for …	Result of Deficiency	Destroyed by …
1	Vitamin A (Retinol)	Liver, fish liver, eggs. cheese, milk products, yellow fruits, chicken	Eyesight, growth, appetite and taste	Night Blindness	Fatty acids
2	Vitamin B1 (Thiamine)	Enriched bread, cereals, liver, pork, whole grains, peanuts, milk	Converting carbohydrates to energy	*Beriberi*: Loss of appetite, weakness, dizziness	High temperatures, alcohol and coffee
3	Vitamin B2 (Riboflavin)	Milk, liver, cheese, leafy vegetables, fish	Helps in metabolism of glucose to produce energy and protein for growth	Itchy, irritation of eyes and mucous membrane	Alcohol and light
4	Vitamin B3 (Niacin)	Green vegetables like peas and green beans, leafy vegetables, milk, fish, cereals, liver	Normal Brain Function, lowers cholesterol and triglyceride levels	*Pellagra*: Loss of memory, lack of concentration, diarrhea, irritability and aggression increases cholesterol	Alcohol, boiling foods and coffee
5	Vitamin B5 (Pantothetic Acid)	Most fruits and vegetables, especially sweet potatoes	Converts fats and carbohydrates to usage energy, aids in reduction of fat	Lack of energy, weakness, tingling and burning feet	Alcohol, coffee
6	Vitamin B6 (Pyridoxine)	Fish, bananas, chicken, port, whole grains	Healthy skin and nervous system, aids in absorption of carbohydrates and protein	Skin inflammation	Alcohol, boiling foods, contraceptive medicines
7	Vitamin B12 (Cobalomin)	Fish, liver, beef, pork, milk, cheese	Making red blood cells	*Pernicious Anemia*: Fatigue, breathing	Water, sunlight, alcohol and

#	Vitamin	Sources	Needed for ...	Result of Deficiency	Destroyed by ...
				Table VI: Essential Vitamins and Their Properties	
				difficulties, dizziness	sleeping pills
8	Vitamin C (Ascorbic Acid)	Citrus fruits, potatoes, berries, green leafy vegetables, peppers	Strengthens immune system, defense against bacteria and viruses, strong laxative, reduces cholesterol	Scurvy: fatigue, bleeding gums, slow healing of damaged tissue and cells	Boiling foods, smoking, light
9	Vitamin D (Calciferol)	Milk, sunlight, tuna, sardines	Healthy bones and teeth	*Rickets*: soften ing of bones and teeth, tooth decay	Mineral oils
10	Vitamin E (Tocopherol)	Nuts, eggs, soybeans, vegetable oils, broccoli, spinach, whole meal products	Fighting toxins in the body	Fat malabsorption, anemia, muscle weakness	Heat, oxygen, chlorine, iron and mineral oils
11	Vitamin K (Menaquinone)	Olive, soybean and Canola oils, broccoli, spinach, mayonnaise	Maintenance of blood platelets	Poor blood clotting, internal bleeding	Anticoagulants, alcohol
12	Folic Acid	Carrots, yeast, liver, eggs, melons, leafy vegetables, rye and whole wheat breads, pumkin	Production of red blood cells	Anemia or low red blood count	Water, sunlight, heat, oestrogen
13	Biotin (Actually a B-Complex vitamin	Egg yolk, liver, leafy vegetables	Healthy cellular growth and maintenance	Hair loss (Alopecia), conjunctivitis, depression, dermatitis	Alcohol

Like vitamins, minerals are needed by the body to assist with metabolism and, like vitamins, minerals are not themselves a source of food. Instead, minerals act like vitamins to support body functions through their interaction with other chemicals in the body. You might think of minerals as the additives in automobile fuels. We must have them, like vitamins, to insure that carbohydrates, proteins and fats are properly and efficiently metabolized. Minerals are essential as mediums and catalysts for efficient chemical reactions needed to convert, for example, carbohydrates to glucose and proteins to amino acids. The four most important minerals required to sustain our bodies are calcium, magnesium, iron and zinc. There are, of course, many other minerals needed by our bodies; but, these four are the most important.

Calcium is extremely important for maintaining the strength and density of bones and teeth and can be derived from milk and milk products like cheeses. Iron is needed for the production and maintenance of red bloods cells and can be derived from eating lean, red meats, oily fish, egg yolks and green leafy vegetables. Magnesium is essential in digestive process, especially for converting carbohydrates to glucose and energy. It is also essential for helping to repair cells and can be derived from eating green leafy vegetables, nuts and whole grain products. Zinc is essential in the efficient metabolism of proteins, fats and carbohydrates and can be derived from most meats, shell fish and whole grains.

5. Water and Fibers

Thus far, we've covered all of the essential nutrients and coenzymes required to actually sustain the healthy state of our bodies. Nevertheless, there are other essential elements needed by the body to survive. Water is clearly an essential element of survival. Without it, the body will dehydrate and wither away like a dried prune. Our bodies have a natural defense mechanism called thirst in order to warn us when our water levels are too low. Water is required to cool our bodies, just like a car radiator, and to carry the nutrients we need to all areas of the body in the form of blood. About 60% of the human body is made up of water of which about 40 ounces per day is expelled through sweat glands and the kidney. Although, we should consume at least 40 ounces of water per day to replace what we lose, this will vary according to physical activity. Just because we need it, it doesn't mean that we should go out and drink five eight-ounce glasses of water. Most of the food we eat contains enormous amounts of water. In fact, about 30% of our water requirements are derived strictly from the foods we eat.

Many of the foods we eat are made up of various substances that we simply cannot digest. For example, much of the content of plants is *cellulose*, a non-digestible component that is used to bond plant cells together, thus giving them their familiar look. Another non-digestible substance is *hemicellulose* which is found in grains like wheat. These non-digestible substances are actually called fibers. Although fibers are non-digestible, they do provide one very valuable function. Because most of the essential nutrients in our body are broken down into small, almost fluid-like matter, that part of this matter that is waste is expelled through the small intestine into the large intestine as fecal waste. Without fiber, this waste would be very soft and mushy. I think that most of us can imagine the rest.

6. Putting it All Together

Having waded through mountains of information about calories, much of it you may think that has nothing to do with obesity, it may help to offer a summary. The illustration at right (Figure 2) gives a general picture of how the foods we eat are divided out and then converted to the components usable by our bodies. Whatever is not used for energy in the form of calories and for the reproduction, repair and maintenance of our cell structure is stored in our bodies as FAT. Although this fat could eventually be used and converted to fuel energy, if it isn't, it will continue to accumulate in our bodies. The illustration also shows how water, minerals, vitamins and fiber are integral parts but not actually directly involved in the production of essential energy. Now that we know fundamentally how our body uses and stores food, we will need to understand the mechanism by which this is actually done.

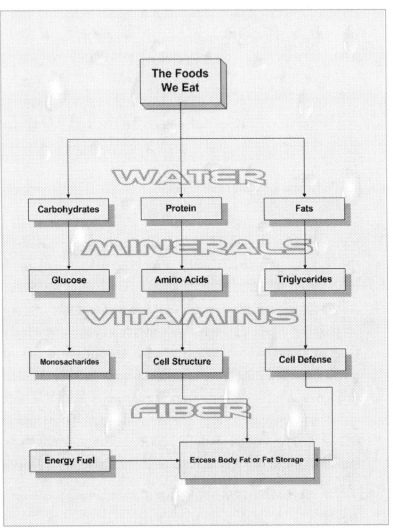

Figure 2: The Digestive Process

C. Metabolism

While physiology refers to the actual mechanical and chemical functions of the body, metabolism refers to how these functions operate. Most of us know basically how a car works and generally most of the many components and chemicals that are required to make it go. We also know that cars operate differently at different speeds, weight, shape and size. The faster the car moves, as a general rule, the more efficiently it will burn fuel. A car also burns more fuel when it accelerates than when it is cruising at a constant speed which is one of the reasons that we get better mileage on the open highway than when driving in a city or town, stopping and accelerating at various stop signs and traffic lights. The heavier a car or truck, the more fuel it will burn per unit of time. It is also true that our cars operate less efficient if their tires are poorly inflated or if we drive erratically and aggressively.

Our bodies have similar properties to that of a car in that some of us burn fuel more efficiently than others and for many, often unrelated reasons. So, two persons of the same body mass can actually eat the same food, but burn it or metabolize it at different rates. If we understand this and the reasons why, it would be much easier to cope with and combat obesity. Of course, the rate at which our bodies burn fuel is measured in calories. As a general rule, the amount of calories that our bodies burn to produce energy is directly proportional to how active we are. Obviously, we burn fewer calories sleeping than we do taking an afternoon stroll around the neighborhood. This is because, at rest, our breathing is slower and shallower, and our heart rate is also slower. What may interest readers is that about 65 percent of the calories we use to burn energy are used exclusively for the operation of our heart, lungs, kidneys and other mechanical functions of the body.

1. How the Body Uses Calories

Since we've already given considerable discussion on the subject of calories one might ask just how many calories would be regarded as normal to sustain our bodies on a typical day. According to the National Institutes of Health and the National Association of Nutritional Sciences, the average, healthy person needs 2,000 calories (kilocalories) each day to survive. This will vary of course depending upon one's age, weight and height, the amount of activity in which the person is engaged and how well the body, for various reasons, will metabolize nutrients. This all translates to the three mechanisms which will determine the amount of calories needed by the body: (1) The Basal Metabolism Rate; (2) Kinetic Metabolism or Activity Metabolism Rate; and, (3) Thermic Metabolism Rate. The number of calories burned by the operation of these three mechanisms will determine how efficiently our bodies convert proteins, carbohydrate and fat to their constituent and usable chemicals in the body.

When a person's body is at rest, age, height and weight will determine this person's *Basal Metabolic Rate* or BMR. The BMR is actually the rate at which an average person metabolizes (or burns) enough fuel to operate the basic life functions of the body, such as breathing, heart beat and kidney functions. One of the most accurate and commonly used measures of the BMR is the Harris-Benedict Formula. This formula is given as follows for both males and females:

$$Males: C = 66 + (6.3 \; x \; W) + (12.9 \; x \; h) - (6.8 \; x \; y)$$

$$Females: C = 665 + (4.3 \; x \; W) + (4.7 \; x \; h) - (4.7 \; x \; y)$$

In these formulas, W = weight in pounds, h = height in inches, y = years of age and C = calories needed. For example, a 55 year-old male, 5 feet, 11 inches tall who weighs 175 pounds will need to burn a minimum of 1,825.9 calories per day as follows:

$$C = 66 + (6.3 \; x \; 175) + (12.9 \; x \; 71) - (6.8 \; x \; 55) = 1,825.9$$

Now, bear in mind that this is only the number of calories required to maintain one's basal metabolism at rest. You may have noticed that age has a significant effect on basal metabolism. In fact, a 20-year-old male of the same weight and height as a 55-year-old will need 244 more calories.

In addition to the calories required for basal metabolism, there are those, of course, needed to support the body when it is engaged in activity. For example, if the individual in the above example goes for a three mile jog, this will require an additional 800 calories. The actual number of calories expended will depend upon the person's weight. The heavier this person is the more calories he/she will need to burn for the same amount of activity because this requires more energy. Certain types of activity can consume more than twice the amount of calories that would be required for basal metabolism. A marathon runner, for example, can burn almost 4.000 calories in this activity alone. **Table VII** below provides of calories burned by weight and commonly engaged activities. Bear in mind that this chart includes only those calories burned at the activities indicated. A more comprehensive activity chart can be found in **Appendix III**.

Table VII: Activity Calories Burned Per Hour			
Activity	**100 lbs**	**150 lbs**	**200 lbs**
Bicycling (12 mph)	210	410	534
Jogging (7 mph)	610	920	1,230
Running (10 mph)	850	1,280	1,664
Swimming (25 yds/min)	185	275	358

Table VII: Activity Calories Burned Per Hour			
Activity	**100 lbs**	**150 lbs**	**200 lbs**
Walking (3 mph)	210	320	416
Walking (4.5 mph)	295	440	572

The calories burned for basal metabolism and physical activity make up about 89% of the amount burned by our bodies on any given day. The remaining 11% is used by the body for the process of actually burning calories. This process includes all of the activities required to convert what we consume to usable energy as described earlier in this chapter. As a general rule, if we add about 10% of the calories required for basal metabolism and physical activity, this would be our total daily fuel requirement. The calories burned to process fuel for energy is called the *thermic effect of food*. Obviously, one must eat food in order to consume the calories necessary to do so. Consequently, the more we eat, the more we will burn for the particular mechanism of body function. This doesn't mean that we should go out and consume a large sausage pizza instead of a bowl of leafy vegetables.

In order to understand what makes us fat, it is important for us also to know the fuel value of foods we eat. We also must know how many calories our bodies need on an average day. This amount is the sum of the calories required for basal metabolism, our usual daily activities, plus the extra 11% needed for the thermic effect. So, using what we've learned thus far, if we need 1,900 calories for basal metabolism, 1,000 calories for what we expect to do in activity each day then we would need another 319 calories for the thermal effect, yielding a total of 3,219 calories per day. Using this number as an example, if we eat and drink 3,500 calories today, our bodies will store the extra 281 calories as fat. With this in mind, suppose we decide, the following day, to only consume 2,938 calories. As logical an approach as this may seem, it will not necessarily work.

Many believe that by starving or fasting in one day to make up for a binge the previous day, everything will be OK. But, what really happens is that, when the body senses starvation, it begins to modify its metabolic engine to compensate. In other words, it goes into starvation mode to survive. In this mode, it actually holds onto the body fat so that it can be released slowly to provide enough energy for long-term survival. This same principal applies to animals, like bears, who build up enormous amounts of fat during most of the year so that enough is available to sustain them in hibernation during the winter months.

Some believe that eating one large meal a day is sufficient to keep one's weight under control. One the contrary, this method actually tends to slow the body's rate of metabolism over time making it even more difficult to lose weight. Remember that the body will always adjust to compensate for our behavior. In fact, it is actually better to consume several small meals per day than one large meal. This also keeps our stomachs from expanding. In fact, eating a large meal actually causes our stomachs to expand and, although it will eventually contract again, this takes a long time. Meanwhile, the larger stomach will make our body think that it is hungry much more frequently as a consequence of its own inherent hunger stimulus.

In addition to eating several smaller rather than one large meal each day, we should also be considerate of the time of the day we choose to eat. Remember that the amount of calories required for basal metabolism is what we burn at rest. With this in mind if we consume more calories than what would be required for basal metabolism shortly before we go to bed at night, all of the excess energy, except that extra 11% needed for digestion, will be stored as fat. Many of us may have heard our parents insist that we should eat at least three meals per day, the largest being the meal we eat at breakfast.

Figure 1 below gives a distribution of calories needed by the body for the functions indicated. These proportions will only vary by a small amount, regardless of the total amount of calories we actually consume each day. For example, if we only consume 2,000 calories, we will use about 1,300 for basal metabolism; however, if we consume 3,000 calories we will use about 1,950 for basal metabolism provided that our activity levels have increased according to our intake. This revelation alone is worthy of note. Suppose now that we consumed 3,000 calories but the number of calories needed for our basal metabolism was still only 1,300. This means that $(1,950 - 1,300) = 650$ calories will be stored as fat.

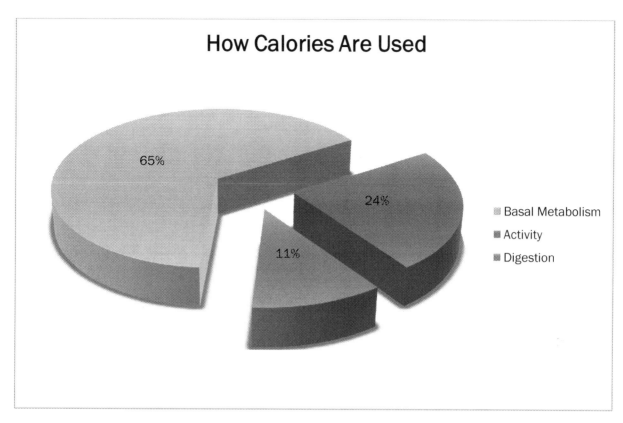

How Calories Are Used

65%

24%

11%

■ Basal Metabolism
■ Activity
■ Digestion

Figure 3: Distribution of calories by body functions

The fact is that the calories needed to energize our basal metabolism, as well as our digestive process, is directly proportional to the amount of activity in which we are engaged. Why? Because when we are more active, our heart rate increases as does our breathing and other bodily functions, accordingly. The more active we are, the more energy will be needed to operate our vital functions. Moreover, the more calories we consume, the more energy will be needed for the digestive process. At rest, we will still use about 65% of the calories we consume for basal metabolism and digestion; hence, any additional calories, including the 24% we would otherwise use when we are active will be stored in the body as fat.

In order to best understand how calories are used, it may be helpful to consider an example. In **Table VIII** below are three individuals each of whom consumes about 3,000 calories per day. One is an Olympic athlete, the second is an active business person and the third is a sedentary retired individual.

Table VIII: Distribution of Usage by Lifestyle for 3,000 Calories Per Day			
Calories Used for ...	Athletic	Average Working	Sedentary
Basal Metabolism	1,950	1,950	1,950
Activity	720	500	100
Digestion	330	330	330
Fat Storage	0	220	620

You should notice in the table that, although the calories used for digestion and basal metabolism are the same, those calories not used for activity, about 24%, are stored as fat. This example is only for illustration purposes because the general metabolism of each of these individuals will vary for a variety of other reasons as we shall explore later in this book.

2. Metabolism and Age

For most of us, the process of actual physical growth occurs between birth and about 25 years of age. During this period, the body's basal metabolic rate is considerably higher because of all the resources required for physical growth. Add to this the fact that most of us at this age are more active, robust and energetic. But, as we get older, our bodies actually begin to get sluggish. This is a combination of a decreased rate of basal metabolism as demonstrated by the Harris-Benedict BMR model described previously and a decrease in physical activity. Although there isn't too much that can be done about the BMR, our physical activity is influenced by many things still within our control. Age usually takes its toll upon us with respect to our ability to perform the activities we did when we were young. Indeed, as we age, so too do our bones and muscles. This in turn affects our general endurance and our ability to engage in the more aggressive activities. Instead of jogging, we may simply walk to prevent injury to our now more brittle bones. Since our reaction times are diminished, our performance in competitive sports like football, baseball and basketball may be replaced by activities such as golf and bicycling.

The fact is that age is clearly an ally of obesity. The older we get, the harder it is to maintain or even lose weight. The reason for this is that our hormone levels begin to decline as we age. In fact, major declines in female progesterone levels and male testosterone levels begin to manifest themselves even at age 35. These important hormones, known as sex hormones, which are especially important in our young adult lives, also have a significant effect upon our basal metabolic rate. The reason we are more active and aggressive as young adults has a large degree to do with the levels of our sex hormones at that age.

3. Effects of Illness and Injury on Metabolism

Just as age can have an impact upon our metabolism so too can illness and injury. In the case of an injury, we become temporarily limited in our mobility or perhaps totally immobile and thus cannot engage in our normal day-to-day activities, at least with the same vigor. In this instance, most of what we consume is used essentially for just rest and thermic metabolism. Consequently, the resumption of our normal dietary habits will likely cause us to gain weight. At the same time, our body needs more energy devoted to the healing process. This tends to offset at least some the potential weight gain.

Unlike an injury which usually does not affect our appetite, an illness such as a cold or flu may render us less active but will also tend to diminish our appetite. Consequently, even though we may be less active, we may actually lose weight. The reason for this is that the body will burn calories in the process of regenerating or repairing cells damaged by infection or by the high temperature of a fever. It should be clear from the previous discussion that proteins are vital for the process of healing because they are the building blocks of cells. Because of the loss of appetite often associated with illness, the body may have to obtain its energy from the fat already stored in the body.

D. Chapter Summary

In order to understand the mechanism of obesity it is essential that we explore the human digestive process and how the foods we eat are used by the body to produce energy. In general, the bulk foods we eat are carried through a network of processes that break them down into matter that can be easily absorbed into the blood stream. The essential nutrients required by our bodies include carbohydrates, proteins and fats. Carbohydrates are converted by digestive hormones to glucose to provide us with energy. Proteins are converted in similar fashion to produce amino acids for cell reproduction and repair. Fats are reduced to triglycerides that are used to protect the cells from damage. Nutrients also carry vitamins and minerals which are used by the body to energize and maintain its hormone balance. Water is essential to provide out bodies with its cooling system and fiber to act as a medium for the transfer of bulk through the body's digestive system.

The food that we eat is processed by the body to produce energy in the form of calories. A calorie is the amount of heat necessary to raise the temperature of one gram of water one degree Celsius. The body needs to burn calories in order to metabolize the food we eat. About 65% of the calories burned from the foods we eat are required for basal metabolism. Basal metabolism consists of the energy required to maintain the body's vital functions such as heart rate, breathing and other organic processes. Another 11% is required by the body to energize the digestive process and the remaining 24% is needed to produce the energy required for daily activities. When the body takes in more nutrients than can be metabolized for these three functional processes, these nutrients are then converted to fat and stored by the body for future use.

What the body cannot metabolize, for whatever reason, is stored as fat. Metabolism will vary from person to person for a multiplicity of reasons, including injury and illness. Age is also a factor contributing to acute changes in metabolism. As the body's ability to metabolize what we eat begins to diminish it is necessary to eat less. Otherwise, the foods we eat which cannot be metabolized will be stored instead as fat.

Key Points:

1. The human body is like a flashlight battery
2. The human body burns nutrients in the form of calories
3. Carbohydrates are converted to glucose to produce energy
4. Proteins are converted to amino acids to replace and/or repair cells
5. Fats are converted to triglycerides to protect cells
6. Vitamins and Minerals are needed by the body to build hormones and digestive chemicals
7. Water provides the body its cooling system
8. Fibers are used by the body as media of waste disposal
9. The rate by which humans burn calories is known as metabolism
10. Metabolism consists of 65% for basic body functions, 11% for digestion and 24% for activity

Chapter 3--*Causes of Obesity*

When most of us think about obesity, perhaps we think of those who eat too much and simply don't exercise like they should. Although this is partially true, it only explains one of the many reasons one can become obese. When the body takes in more nutrients than it can burn off, these nutrients are stored as adipose tissue or fat. It is clear that our bodies need nourishment to survive. The food we eat is burned, like the fuel in a car, as it is used by our bodies to do basically what we do day after day. Sometimes the body needs more fuel than other times. We burn much more fuel, or put more scientifically, use more energy standing than we do sleeping and much more walking than we do standing and so on. The more energy we burn the more fuel (or food) we will need for our bodies to remain within a normal body mass.

It is very important to understand that no one individual ever expends the same amount of fuel as another even while performing the same activities. In fact, there are numerous factors that will determine how much fuel an individual will burn per unit of time. These factors include age, basal metabolism, genetic predisposition, gender, psychological profile, environment and even social and cultural origin. Two individuals of the same height, weight, body frame, age, and so on, both jogging together at the same rate will still burn fuel at different rates depending upon their metabolism. Most of us have known someone in our lives who can eat voraciously and yet not gain weight and someone else who eats very little yet suffers with chronic weight problems. In this chapter, we will explore the many causes of obesity, some of which may be surprising.

As a general rule, despite the many factors that may prevail against our quest to remain within the normal range of body mass, there is no hard evidence that disputes the fact that the more we eat and/or the less we exercise, the more weight we will gain. If we don't burn the fuel that results from what we eat or drink, it will just continue to accumulate in our bodies in the form of adipose tissue—FAT. So, the old adage that diet and exercise are essential in maintaining fitness is quite true, but for various reasons that will be made clear later in this book some individuals actually must eat less and exercise more than others, and that is what has become the source of much consternation, mountains of clinical research and a litany of diet fads, many of them disreputable, that seem to permeate society. Then there are those who actually believe that exercise is not at all necessary if you just eat the right foods. Still others believe that we can eat as much as we want as long as it's a little bit at a time during each day.

We all know that what and how much we eat will determine what we are physically. If this is indeed so, then you would expect that how we appear is completely under our control. In other words, you would think that all we need to do to remain a perfect weight all of our lives is to regulate our eating habits. Right? Not so fast! Since we've already indicated that no two persons will metabolize food the same way, it is clear that some other, perhaps many other factors, will have an influence upon how we develop physically. For this reason, if and when we get fat, it is probably not all our fault in all cases. Instead, we may be up against a "stacked deck" of reasons over which we have little or perhaps absolutely no control.

A. Psychosocial Causes of Obesity

Among the most significant causes of obesity are those that are bundled into that complex web of actions which are influenced largely by our own behavior and the social conventions of the community in which we live. The way we behave as individuals is a function of how we perceive our environment and certainly how we believe we ourselves are perceived. There is a wide array of psychosocial factors that can cause us to be fat, but not all of these factors are necessarily under our control even if we concentrate. Certainly a big psychosocial factor contributing to obesity is lack of exercise coupled with a tendency to overeat. But this is often influenced by many other conditions, including our own personality, our environment, the rigors and time-constraints associated with our jobs as well as well as the many untoward habits we may have acquired, such as excessive alcohol consumption, smoking and drug abuse and, in general, our life style.

1. Lifestyles

The way that we live our daily lives, what, where, when and how we eat and, of course, what we do and how we do it will to a great extent determine how we look and feel. This bundle of factors is rolled into a pattern of behavior called our lifestyle. Our lifestyle is basically what we do regularly everyday from the time we wake up until we go to bed. A typical lifestyle may include an early morning walk, followed by breakfast, a drive to work, afternoon lunch, more work, late afternoon drink or two, dinner, a couple of hours of TV and then on to bed again. Although perhaps mundane, this is actually just one of many different lifestyles into which we each entrench ourselves. By entrenched, I mean that it actually becomes a habit, like smoking, that is often very difficult to overcome.

In general, there are three types of lifestyles: (1) Active-Aggressive, (2). Passive-Aggressive, (3) Passive-Sedentary. In the active-aggressive category will be most professional athletes and those who exercise two to four hours each day. Although this category consists of those with highly active lifestyles, obesity may still prevail for those who consume more than their bodies need even for their intense activities. Indeed, those with highly active lifestyles tend to have larger appetites and thus must watch their caloric intake very carefully. The passive-aggressive lifestyle is the one in which most of us will fall. In this lifestyle, we may exercise less than one hour per day, but our daily activities from work and the things we do at home make up for this. Nevertheless, this category consists of a majority of those who are considered overweight, but not necessarily obese. Those in this category who are obese tend to allow their activities to interfere with good or acceptable eating habits. In the passive-sedentary category are those who do not exercise at all and engage in very little if any activity. Those in this category you might classify as the quintessential "couch potatoes". In fact, the passive-sedentary lifestyle consists almost entirely of overweight and obese individuals. Nevertheless, these do not necessarily include individuals whose lifestyles are compelled by disabilities or illnesses.

In the active-aggressive category, obesity is rare because individuals in this category are not only very active, but they tend to eat according to strict guidelines and on diets that are best suited to the physical activities in which they are engaged. Despite this, however, those in the active-aggressive category are considerably more in danger of becoming obese than those in the passive-aggressive category. The reason for this is quite alarming. When an individual spends years in an active-aggressive lifestyle then very suddenly retires or relaxes into the passive-aggressive or passive-sedentary lifestyle, his/her customary eating habits tend to fall prey to a substantially reduced basal metabolism. This is much like going into an alcoholic or drug withdrawal state.

Those in the passive-aggressive lifestyle are also dangerously predisposed to obesity, but not so much from changes in their basal metabolism. Instead, they tend to fall prey to their own busy schedules. Those who are active in everything else but exercise tend to have much less time to plan and prepare healthy meals. These individuals will tend to eat out more and, in far too many cases, at the so called "fast food" establishments where meals are preprocessed and very high in calories.

The passive-sedentary lifestyle is consistent with individuals who, for various reasons, remain largely inactive. Many of these individuals are unable to engage in activity for health reasons, because they may be physically handicapped or may be too old to engage in physical activities safely. Those in this category are also drop-outs from the other two categories because they became obese and may be far too overweight to conjure the energy for physical activity.

2. Personality Traits

The reader may wonder how someone's personality could have anything to do with obesity. Well, you see, how we are as individuals is directly proportional to how we behave. For example, highly competitive and aggressive individuals tend to participate actively in sports and, for this reason, would be less likely to become obese. On the other hand, individuals who have a so called "laid-back" and relaxed personality tend to be less active and thus more likely to become obese. In the early 1950's, a nine-year study conducted by cardiologists, Meyer

Freidman and R. H. Rosenman revealed two distinct personality types and their links to obesity and heart disease. Derived from this study was a theory that distinguished the general profile of individuals between a **Type A** and a **Type B** personality.

Based on this theory of personality types, a Type A personality was descriptive of someone with highly competitive and aggressive tendencies. Type A individuals are restless, time-conscious and status-oriented. Their nature tends to make it difficult for them to relax; hence, they are always active and often impatient. As a consequence of their personality profile, Type A individuals tend to become stressed and anxious and thus more prone to developing high-risk medical conditions such as hypertension and cardiovascular disease. Despite this, however, Type A individuals are not very likely to become obese. The reason for this is that they are usually very active and indeed, very self-conscious of how they are perceived. As a matter of clinical study, when a Type A individual becomes obese it is more the consequence of metabolism and underlying disease than of lifestyle; however, Type A individuals tend to become more prone to alcohol and drug abuse, behavior that itself can result in obesity.

By contrast to that of a Type A personality, the Type B individual is generally relaxed and non-aggressive and lacking any sense of urgency. Type B individuals tend to take life in stride and are generally very well-liked for this reason. Unlike the Type A individuals, however, those with Type B personalities tend to procrastinate and are often disorganized and out of focus. Type B individuals usually have a very high self-esteem, therefore, despite their organizational shortcomings, tend to advance faster and more lucratively in their careers. Type B individuals also tend to be far less active and competitively aggressive than their Type A counterparts and for this reason, tend to become obese. In this case, the tendency for obesity among Type B individuals is almost invariably related to lifestyle.

3. Alcohol, Drug Abuse and Smoking

It is interesting to note with respect to the previous discussion on personality types that Type A individuals are more likely than Type B individuals to take alcohol and drugs. The reason for this is that they view this as a way of overcoming stress, anxiety and lack of self-esteem. Unfortunately, these activities cannot only cause serious medical conditions, but also obesity. Alcohol abuse is sort of a double-edged sword because if its consumption doesn't contribute to obesity, it can otherwise result in nutritional deficiencies. The reason for this is that individuals who consume alcohol tend to also eat less to avoid becoming obese. With drugs, there are even more dangerous manifestations, but not necessarily those directly attributable to the development of obesity. Instead, drugs tend to upset a person's metabolism in ways that make the body less efficient at digesting food. Drugs also tend to cause changes in behavior that may affect the eating habits of those who abuse them.

Although alcohol taken in small or moderate quantities may actually bear health benefits, too much alcohol can cause obesity. For Type A individuals, small amounts of alcohol taken daily are known to reduce stress and thus also reduce the likelihood of heart disease. But large and frequent amounts of alcohols intake, while certainly a major contributor of liver and heart disease, in and of itself, can cause obesity. Alcohol is very high in calories. When we drink alcohol it is generally a blend of substances that are naturally fermented to produce ethanol or ethyl alcohol. Although ethyl alcohol is high in sugar and carbohydrate content, it has very little if any food value. Ethyl alcohol is actually metabolized by the body as acetate to produce energy; however, it contains no vitamins, minerals or protein. Moreover, consumption of alcohol can actually induce an appetite. It can also increase the rate at which we store fat. The reason for this is that alcohol metabolizes more efficiently than most foods. During the process of metabolizing alcohol, the oxidation of fat is significantly reduced. Because alcohol actually hinders the oxidation of fat, the latter will remain it in the body accordingly.

With drug abuse, an even more complex and insidious outcome can result in obesity. A chemical in the brain which helps to regulate our appetite is called *dopamine*. Studies have actually demonstrated that drugs such as heroin and cocaine will diminishes the levels of dopamine necessary to control certain feelings such as sexual arousal and gratification from food. Consequently, this may result in a range of excessive compulsive behaviors, including an increased appetite for food. Marijuana is a drug well known for its tendency to increase human appetite. Those who smoke marijuana frequently tend to become obese resulting from the immediate and often severe fits of hunger that results from smoking this substance.

While on the subject of smoking, many believe that smoking tobacco actually helps to control appetite and thus can prevent the onset of obesity. To a certain extent, this is true; however, smoking accomplishes this by increasing the basal metabolism rate. When someone smokes a cigarette this increases both the heart rate and respiration, two body functions that require energy for basal metabolism. Because smokers tend to take cigarettes regularly all throughout the day, during the intervening times between meals, the additional energy required for the higher basal metabolic rate will be taken from any excess fat that is stored in the body. Even though the mechanism of smoking can actually help to control the onset of obesity, much in the way that other drugs reduce the levels of dopamine in the brain so too does nicotine. Consequently, many individuals that smoke develop increased appetites and eventually become obese despite the metabolic benefits of this habit. More importantly, obesity is especially prevalent among individuals who quit smoking after having prevailed in this behavior for many years.

4. Career-Related Causes of Obesity

In the fast-pace world of modern business, our biggest enemy is now time—time to relax, to exercise and to best manage our personal lives. Today, it is not enough for just one member of the family to become gainfully employed. More than ever before in history, both married spouses will have jobs and, in many cases, merely to make ends meet economically. If not married, it is likely that individuals work longer hours or perhaps even more than one job in order to either survive financially or to maintain a chosen lifestyle. In either case, the time required to effectively manage the dietary and health needs of our body is significantly impaired. Instead of having the time to prepare a healthy and properly proportioned and apportioned meal, we tend to obtain our meals more frequently at the so called "fast food" restaurants or, for that matter, any restaurant. Even if we are careful to order diet conscious meals, restaurants will usually prepare them to both tease and please the palette. Restaurant meals are generally prepared from food rich with preservatives and stylish cuisines rich in salt, sugar and other spices for taste.

In addition to the way careers can hinder our ability to prevent obesity our choice of career can also be a pre-determinant of obesity. Generally, most white-collar jobs, such as those that are administrative, professional and clerical in nature require that we sit at a desk during most of the work day. This is consistent with a passive-aggressive lifestyle. Many conscientious white-collar employers now offer exercise programs and more frequent rest periods to help combat obesity in the work place. But, this is done primarily to reduce their exposure to workers compensation claims and higher group insurance premiums if they offer health insurance benefits.

By contrast to the more sedentary nature of the white-collar careers, blue-collar, semi-skilled and industrial jobs tend to be very active. Most of these jobs include those that demand heavy lifting and hard work in general such as construction, maintenance and cleaning jobs. But some blue-collar jobs can also be quite sedentary, especially those in the transportation industry such as truck, taxi, bus and limousine drivers. Police and fire fighters are especially prone to obesity as a direct function of what they are required to do in their jobs. Unlike in the early days when police officers would "walk a beat" so to speak, in modern times they tend to operate from a police car or cruiser most of the day. Firefighters spend the lion's share of each day waiting for a fire alarm. Although much of this idle time is spent in training activities it is still not sufficient to make this an active-aggressive career choice.

With many careers the challenges of the work place can impose an inordinate amount of stress upon the employee. In modern times, the stress associated with career growth has become more and more overcome by the stress associated simply with holding a job. Stress in the work place contributes significantly to the onset of obesity and for many reasons. Stress can upset the body's immune system. Stress can also lead to depression and anxiety, alcoholism, drug abuse and a generally repressed life style all of which can contribute to obesity.

5. Depression and Anxiety

It is likely that people who are already overweight are also depressed about their condition, but while depression can be a consequence of obesity it can also be a cause. Just as drug abuse can reduce the level of dopamine in the brain, so too can chemical imbalances resulting, for example, from pregnancy and menopause in women and reduced vitality in men. Dopamine not only regulates our appetite and sex drive, it also helps to regulate how we feel emotionally—our state of happiness or sadness. Consequently, when there is a metabolically induced reduction of dopamine in the brain, we will not only become depressed but concurrently will tend to have more robust appetites. This in turn can cause obesity. But this is only part of the cause. In fact, depression can actually be controlled by overeating. Imagine that! So, we're depressed, we eat more and then suddenly we begin to feel better emotionally. Why? Well, one of the consequences of depression is the activation of the *endocannabinoid system* (ECS).

The ECS is a complex set of molecules in the central and peripheral nervous system that help to regulate and control pain, mood, appetite and memory. The ECS is actually fed by amino acids metabolized from protein. Episodes of depression occur when the ECS is chemically or metabolically suppressed from a reduction in amino acids. This in turn triggers the ECS receptors that control appetite to demand more protein. Coincidentally, the resulting increase in appetite becomes in fact therapeutic because when we eat this then restores the necessary amino acids and thus brings the ECS back in balance thereby at least temporarily eliminating our depressed state. Unfortunately, the therapeutic treatments for depression over time can result in obesity.

Yet another ally of obesity is anxiety. Anxiety is an obsessive-compulsive state that causes the body to produce more adrenaline. An overproduction of adrenaline will require more nutrients in the form of glucose. This in turn will increase our appetites and thus lead potentially to obesity. Although the link between obesity and anxiety is not clearly understood, scientists generally agree that mood changes are controlled in the brain as are the receptors that control appetite. Scientists do not necessarily agree on the mechanisms which cause or trigger anxiety. Many believe that anxiety is a function of the environment, social conventions, economic conditions and other factors which may pose threats upon our livelihood. These same factors also contribute to depression, suicidal tendencies and other mental health problems. What scientists cannot agree upon is whether or not anxiety is chemical or behavioral. The former may be treated by drugs, but the latter requires long-term therapeutic counseling.

6. What and How We Eat

Although there have been reports of overweight persons actually eating less than individuals of normal weight, one thing that should go without saying is that we simply can't get fat without eating something. In most cases, it's not necessarily just the food itself which can cause obesity. In fact, the principal cause of obesity from overeating is linked to the structure of our diet, when and how often we eat. Earlier in this book, we indicated that about 24% of the calories we consume are burned during whatever activities in which we are engaged. The key word here is "activity". If we eat and do not actively burn what we eat, the body will store it. Having said this then, it is important to understand that the time of day during which we eat is equally as important as what we eat. In terms of what we eat, we know that some foods have more calories than others. In fact, we can actually consume an ounce of one type of food having two to three times as many calories as four ounces of another kind. A large bowl of salad, for example, may have just as many calories as a single bite of cheese cake, but the latter will likely not be enough to satisfy our appetites.

In **Chapter 2**, a considerable amount of discussion prevailed on the subject of calories and how they are metabolized in the body. It was noted that the rate of metabolism per hour is certainly dependent upon the activities in which we are engaged. It was also noted that when an individual goes for hours without eating, the body will think that it is starving and lower its metabolism accordingly. For example, those who eat just one meal per day will have a much lower metabolism than those who eat several meals each day. Even if we do eat just one meal each day, our potential for becoming obese will depend upon the time of day at which we eat such a meal. Because we are active from the time we get up in the morning until we go back to sleep at night, it is only logical to suggest we should eat our one meal in the morning or just after we wake up. If we eat instead just before going to bed, because our bodies are at rest, the lower resulting metabolism will substantially increase our potential for becoming obese. Moreover, the process of digestion will tend to increase the level of adrenaline in the body thus contributing to restlessness.

As a general rule, although not scientifically conclusive, we should not eat just one meal per day. Rather than eating one large meal, especially if this is shortly before we go to bed at night, we should eat several smaller meals, the largest of these being as soon after we awake as practical. By consuming several smaller meals per day, our body will scarcely have the time to think that we are in starvation mode. Most dieticians and dietary consultants will recommend three balanced meals each day, the largest of which should be consumed for breakfast. But most of us behave quite the contrary, perhaps eating a bagel for breakfast, a sandwich for lunch and then a large meal a couple of hours before we go to sleep. One problem with eating large meals is that they tend to stretch our stomachs. As this is done, after several hours, the larger unoccupied space in the stomach can induce hunger pangs.

7. Social Convention

Suppose for the sake of illustration that we were born to a society of obese individuals? In fact, everyone around us, including our loved ones, is obese and this is how they remain throughout life. Because we are literally surrounded by a society of obese individuals this now is our only frame of reference to how we should appear. Consequently, we will become obese by the process of social convention. By social convention, I mean the group behavior, attitude and general lifestyles of an entire community or society. Since we simply can't escape the conventions of society, we must assimilate with it or become socially outcast.

The influence of culture and society upon our own behavior is a powerful and inescapable force. In fact, the ways of a society will actually form the lifetime patterns of our own behavior, including how and what we eat, how and what we wear and basically how we behave each day. In short, as they say, "When in Rome, do as the Romans do." Because culture and society is a major influence on behavior and lifestyles a considerable amount will be addressed on this subject in **Section II** of this book.

8. Food Addiction

Just as alcohol, tobacco and narcotic drugs can be addictive, scientists have determined that food itself can be addictive as well. Indeed, the psychological makeup of certain individuals may predispose them to a type of obsessive behavior known as *hedonic hunger.* It is believed that those who suffer from hedonic hunger react voraciously to the sight and smell of foods. In normal individuals, hunger is controlled by the hormone leptin which is released to control appetite. This normal activity is referred to as homeostatic hunger. In those who suffer from hedonic hunger obsession, on the other hand, the production of leptin is somehow overcome by an overproduction of dopamine. Recall that dopamine is released in reaction to the brain activity involving memory, thinking, emotion and reward.

B. Medical Causes of Obesity

Thus far, we have offered extensive discussion upon the many factors that can influence the onset of obesity even to the point of assuring ourselves that lack of exercise and overeating cannot always be the cause of obesity. In fact, there are so many reasons why we gain weight that adherence to a strict diet and even vigorous exercise cannot always prevent it. A major reason for this can be attributed to underlying medical conditions such as hypothyroidism, Cushing's Disease, metabolic syndrome and others.

1. Hyperthyroidism and Hypothyroidism

One of the largest and most important endocrine glands in the body is the thyroid gland. Situated at the base of the neck just below the thyroid cartilage or "Adams Apple", the thyroid gland actually regulates how quickly the body uses energy. In other words, the thyroid gland controls the metabolic functions of the body. This means that our basal metabolism, which we discussed in Chapter 2, is dependent on the thyroid gland for its proper function. The thyroid gland also regulates growth and development from birth to maturity and signals the body to stop growing at around age 25.

A normal thyroid gland produces two hormones, *thyroxin (T4)* and *triiodothyronine (T3)*. The T4 hormone is used by the thyroid gland to stimulate the body's consumption of oxygen and thus the metabolism of cells and tissue through the production of iodine. In fact, T4 stands for 4 atoms of iodine and T3, 3 atoms of iodine. About 80% of the hormones produced in the thyroid gland consist of the T4 hormone and 20% of the T3 hormone. Despite its capacity in comparison to the T4 hormone, the T3 hormone, which is produced by or converted from the T4 hormone, actually does the lion's share of the work at activating and regulating the body's metabolism.

The point to all of this technical talk is that when more or less of the T4 and T3 hormones are produced, a number of conditions can become manifest. Among these is a condition known as *hyperthyroidism*. Hyperthyroidism is the term used to describe an overactive thyroid or a thyroid that produces too much T4 and/or T3. Although this condition tends to accelerate the body's metabolic rate it does so at a significant cost. Indeed, while hyperthyroidism actually increases the rate by which the body burns calories, this in turn increases appetite, almost to the point of inducing voracious hunger. As a result, some patients with hyperthyroidism can gain weight. Adding to this is the fact that hyperthyroidism can cause muscle weakness and fatigue thus significantly reducing the body's ability to stay active. Those with hyperthyroidism can also feel very hot, often irritable and easily agitated. Hyperthyroidism can also contribute to many other predispositions for obesity, including depression and anxiety, insomnia and impaired mental and physical ability.

Although *HYPER*thyroidism can cause weight gain from an increase in appetite, *HYPO*thyroidism causes weight gain regardless of appetite. In fact, hypothyroidism is more associated with obesity than hyperthyroidism. With hypothyroidism, the thyroid gland produces too little of the T4 and/or T3 hormones thus actually resulting in a decrease in metabolism. This is caused primarily by an inflammation of the thyroid gland resulting from a deficiency in the body's immune system, a condition known as autoimmune thyroiditis or Hashimoto's thyroiditis.

Unlike hyperthyroidism, hypothyroidism does not have a direct relationship to appetite because the body's need for nourishment to sustain basic bodily functions is still necessary; thus, while hyperthyroidism may cause an increase in appetite, hypothyroidism does not necessarily bring about a decrease in appetite as one might expect. Symptoms of hypothyroidism are similar to those of hyperthyroidism, but can also include an enlargement of the thyroid gland, a condition known as goiter. Goiters are caused from a deficiency of iodine.

Approximately 10 million Americans and about 4% of the general population suffer from hypothyroidism which appears to occur mostly in women, especially elderly woman. Because of the diminished metabolism resulting from hypothyroidism, weight gain is generally predisposed with this condition. Left untreated, hypothyroidism can lead to morbid obesity, severe depression, heart disease and coma.

2. Cushing's Disease

When the body is under stress, there are many hormones released to protect it from harm. For example, adrenalin is released by the adrenal glands to increase the body's strength, endorphin is released by the pituitary glands to induce shock or control pain when we are injured, and a hormone known as cortisol is released also by the adrenal glands to help the body cope with stress. Cortisol coincidentally also regulates blood sugar levels in the body by counteracting any overproduction of insulin during the digestive process. You may recall from Chapter 2 that blood sugar or glucose is converted from carbohydrates to heat energy or calories. You should recall also that insulin is produced by the pancreas in order to regulate the amount of glucose that is transferred into our cells. If too much insulin is produced, this will result in a decrease in blood sugar. But if too little insulin is produced then blood sugar levels will rise and this is precisely what happens when the body produces too much cortisol.

Although increased levels of cortisol can occur as a result of a hormone disorder in the adrenal glands, it can also result from an overuse of steroids. Steroids are used extensively by patients suffering from asthma, arthritis and those with muscle inflammation. The long-term overproduction or saturation of cortisol can result in a condition known as *hypercortisolism*, more commonly referred to as Cushing's Syndrome. The most obvious symptom of Cushing's Syndrome is upper body obesity manifested by puffy cheeks and an enlarged neck. Cushing's Syndrome results primarily from a diminished metabolism of glucose and is very common in those having Type 2 diabetes.

Cushing's Syndrome is often associated with individuals under stress from illness, injury or certain lifestyle choices. Because higher than normal levels of cortisol are released during stressful periods, those who suffer from long-term anxiety and depression, as well as alcoholics and drug abusers, may tend to develop the disease. The reason for this is that increased levels of cortisol are released to help regulate breathing and heart rate, both of which are elevated during stress. Long-term stress can make the body think that more cortisol is needed for cardiovascular functions. It is interesting to note that when the cardiovascular system is over-regulated this can result in the onset of hypertension (high blood pressure).

3. Polycystic Ovary Syndrome (PCOS)

While high levels of cortisol can cause obesity, most notably from an over-regulation of insulin, low levels of cortisol can result in an over production of insulin. High levels of insulin in the body are thought to result in an increase in the hormone *androgen* which can cause obesity in females, especially in and around the area of the hip. Androgen, by the way, is a hormone released both in males and females. In addition to weight gain, high levels of androgen can also cause excessive hair growth, acne and problems with ovulation. High levels of androgen in females can lead to a condition known as Policystic Ovary Syndrome (PCOS). PCOS is an endocrine disorder that affects about 5% to 10% of females, especially those of reproductive ages 15 through 46. Though PCOS can lead to infertility in females, there is also a strong correlation between this syndrome and obesity. In fact, although the relationship between PCOS and obesity are not clearly understood, approximately 50% of woman who suffer from PCOS are obese.

So, there just doesn't seem to be too many ways around this problem of obesity especially when there is an imbalance of one or more hormones in the body.

4. Metabolic Syndrome

An imbalance of hormones for any reason can lead to a variety of adverse conditions, including obesity. Any hormone imbalance, physical or psychosocial predisposition which limits or significantly changes the normal metabolic actions of the body, including basal metabolism, activity metabolism, and thermic metabolism can result in a collection of physiological states known as metabolic syndrome. Metabolic syndrome is both a cause and an effect of obesity. When metabolic syndrome is a cause of obesity it is usually the result of aging, injury or disease. But metabolic syndrome can also result from the body's resistance to insulin, a sedentary lifestyle, a diet too high in carbohydrates, alcoholism and even smoking. In general, metabolic syndrome is the collection of factors that result in a deficiency of the body's ability to metabolize food or burn calories. As a result, those having the condition can develop abdominal obesity, the so called, "beer belly", insulin resistance, hypertension (high blood pressure) and a predisposition to cardiovascular disease. As will be addressed in the next chapter, metabolic syndrome can be a precursor of Type 2 diabetes when associated obesity.

5. Other Medical Causes of Obesity

Although the primary medical causes of obesity have already been covered there are dozens of other medical conditions that can cause obesity, but not necessarily to the same extent. Rather than to inundate the reader with a detailed explanation of these diseases, these, as well as the ones discussed previously in this chapter, are summarized along with their clinical description in **Table IV** below.

Table IX: Medical Causes of Obesity		
Disease	**Description**	**Symptoms**
Hypothyroidism	Inflammation of the thyroid gland resulting in underproduction of thyroid hormones that regulate metabolism	Abnormal weight gain, iodine insufficiency and possible goiter
Cushing's Disease	Overproduction of cortisol from long-term exposure to corticosteroids (steroids)	Increase in blood sugar, decrease in insulin, puffy cheeks, upper body obesity
Polycystic Ovary Disease	Overproduction of androgen hormone in females	Increase in size of hips, disrupted ovulation
Metabolic Syndrome	Reduction in metabolism resulting from age, injury and/or disease	Abnormal weight gain, "beer belly"
Laurence-Moon-Biedl Syndrome	Hereditary condition resulting in multiple disorders, including hypogonadism, retinitis and paraplegia	Mental retardation, abnormal body stature and weight gain
Hyperandrogenism	Similar to polycystic ovary disease in that it results from excessive levels of androgen in females	Abnormal weight gain, excessive body hair in females, deepening of voice, irregular menstrual cycle
Pituatary Gland Disease		
Prader-Willis Syndrome	A rare chromosome disorder resulting from a misprinted DNA	Abnormal weight gain, mental retardation
Klinefelter Syndrome	A genetic condition resulting from too many x and y chromosomes during cell division	Abnormal skeletal and sexual development, breast enlargement in males, obesity
Idiopathic Edema	A condition of unknown (idiopathic) cause resulting in an abnormal	Fluid retention, facial, feet and hand

Table IX: Medical Causes of Obesity		
__Disease__	__Description__	__Symptoms__
	retention of sodium	swelling
Sohlar-Soffer Syndrome	A rare disease of unknown etiology (cause) that results in mental retardation and acute skeletal disorders	Fasting hyperglycemia, glucose intolerance, hypogonadism, abnormal weight gain, abnormal bone development
Hypergonadism	Under-activity of the gonads (ovaries and testes)	Lack of facial hair, decreased testicular volume, short stature, abnormal weight gain
MOMO Syndrome	A rare birth defect resulting in abnormal weight and shape at birth	Enlarged skull, childhood obesity
HAIR-AN Syndrome	A rare disease in females characterized by insulin resistance and an over-abundance of male hormones	Hypertension, increased libido, glucose intolerance, deep voice, abnormal weight gain, irregular menstrual cycle
Achard-Theirs Syndrome	Post menopausal Diabetes Mellitus and hirsuitism (excessive hair growth)	Abnormal weight gain, deepening voice, excessive body hair
Cholicystitis (Gallbladder Disease)	Gall stones formed from bile containing too much cholesterol	Severe abdominal pain, heartburn, belching, abnormal weight gain
Reidel Syndrome	Excessive growth of fibrous tissue around thyroid area resulting in the latter's eventual destruction	Difficulty breathing, hoarseness, swallowing difficulty, abnormal weight gain
Frolich's Syndrome	An endocrine abnormality resulting from tumors or damage to the hypothalamus	Retarded sexual development, large hips, fatty breast growth before puberty, obesity

C. Heredity

In **Figure I** on Page 33, you may have noticed that the lion's share or about 65% of the calories we need each day are used just for basal metabolism or for the functions of our vital organs when we are at rest. Another 11% is used for the mechanics of digestion leaving a scant 24% that is really under our immediate control. You may wonder then how we can get fat. Well, a big part of the answer rests within the complex array of our genetic profile. You see, some cars drive better than others. Some get better gas mileage than others and some can accelerate and break better than others and it's all a function of how they are made. With this in mind, the efficiency by which we burn calories, even for basal metabolism, really depends upon just how well we're made. How we're made depends upon our genetic makeup.

Genetics is a complex array of processes that basically determine how we will develop as a human organism. When we think of genetics, we are referring to our DNA (deoxyribonucleic acid). Our DNA is sort of like the blue print to an architectural structure and is thus used to determine just how we will become who we are. Our DNA structure is more commonly referred to as our genes. Genes are the links (or pages in a history book) that tie us to our lineage, including our parents, grandparents, great grandparents and all the way back to our earliest ancestors. Within the makeup of our genes are markers of information accumulated by the behavior and physical development of our heritage.

Studies have shown that a strong link exists between heredity and obesity. According to these studies, most of the respondents surveyed who were themselves obese had either one or both parents who were also obese. While studies may suggest that we are "Like father, like son" or "like mother, like daughter" perhaps, this could also be the result of how our parents may have influenced our eating habits or general behavior. Nevertheless, studies have actually been conducted that involved identical twins who were separated and raised by different families and both of whose parents were obese. As it turns out, in most cases, each of the twins became themselves obese, even under the influence of different familial behavior and dietary habits. These results suggest a genetic link to obesity.

Recently, studies in genetics have isolated a so-called "fat gene" that may be the precursor of our development into obesity. This gene is appropriately called the Ob gene (short for obesity). Scientists believe that the gene evolved from the behavior of early tribal cultures whose tendency to store fat was likely the result of frequent and extended periods of severe famine. The Ob gene is often called the "thrifty gene" in that it tends to make us think we are hungry even after the body is sufficiently full and well-nourished. This is thought to be caused by the production of a deficient variant of a protein called leptin. In normal individuals, leptin is actually a chemical that signals the brain when our stomachs are full and that we should therefore stop eating. The leptin receptor that is produced by the Ob gene is believed to be defective and thus may underestimate when we are no longer hungry.

Heredity is less an influence on obesity if it is merely a function of behavior than a function of the various diseases or metabolic conditions that cause obesity. In other words, just because our parents may have had a tendency to overeat, this does not necessarily mean that we will inherit (or more appropriately, acquire) that type of behavior. Indeed, parents are a major influence upon our lives as children; however, as we mature and move independently into the real world, our behavior is then influenced by many other things including job, personal and professional relationships and other factors we introduced in our discussion of the psychosocial causes of obesity.

Disease and metabolic profile are physiological processes whose mechanism is a function of genetic design. By disease, I am referring, of course, to those that are autonomous and not acquired or contagious. An autonomous disease or condition is one that occurs in the body without any known external or environmental cause. Acquired and contagious diseases are not known to be genetically transferred hereditarily. An acquired disease is one that is induced by exposure to a substance, chemical or process in the environment. Examples of acquired diseases include skin cancer from exposure to the sun, cancer or emphysema from smoking, alcoholic liver disease and so on. Contagious diseases are those derived from contact with airborne or blood borne viruses and pathogens.

1. Heredity as a Factor of Psychosocial Behavior

Many of the psychosocial causes of obesity discussed previously may actually have a genetic basis. Although scientists are not entirely in agreement on this, there are certain human traits which may impose a genetic predisposition to obesity. For example, those who drink alcohol, those who smoke or those who abuse drugs can actually pass these habits on to their offspring, even without any social influence. The primary reason for this is based upon the addictive properties of these substances. For example, women who smoke or abuse drugs and alcohol during pregnancy can give birth to a child already predisposed with this addiction. The reason for this is that the addictive properties of the abused substance are transmitted through the blood stream of the unborn child.

Studies have shown that by comparison to those who are not, children born to alcoholic parents are more likely to become alcoholics themselves. This is true also of smokers and drug abusers. Although these studies point to a genetic trend, scientists have yet to isolate a specific gene that may pass these traits on to offspring and are convinced that there may be many genes involved. But most scientists readily agree that addiction and parental influence rather than genetics may be the predisposing transmitter of this behavior.

Studies have also shown that heredity plays a significant factor in the development of one's personality. Behavioral geneticists at the George Washington University under Dr. David Reiss have conducted extensive research which points to one's personality as being genetically predisposed. These studies have shown that if the dominant parent is a Type A personality, this trait will likely pass to the offspring, even if the other parent is a Type B personality. Recall that persons having a Type B personality are more likely to become overweight or obese than those with a Type A personality.

2. Heredity as a Factor of Medical Condition

Many of the diseases that can cause obesity can also be genetically transmitted to the offspring and the precarious drama continues. Common among these are Prader-Willis syndrome and Bardet-Beidle syndrome. Although these are rare conditions, they both predispose their victims to obesity. Prader-Willis syndrome (PWS) is a genetic condition characterized by multiple abnormal states including hypotonia (short stature), small hands and feet, hypogonadism, behavioral issues, mild mental retardation and, of course, obesity, especially around the lower abdomen. The cause of obesity in patients with PWS is usually a result of an excessively abnormal appetite caused by an overabundance of the hormone ghrelin. This is one of the hormones released to regulate appetite, but too much of this hormone will actually cause an increase in one's appetite even if the body is fully nourished. Bardet-Beidle Syndrome (BBS) is another rare genetic disorder that can cause obesity. Symptoms of BBS are similar to those of PWS; however, the actually mechanism of its influence on obesity is not clearly understood. It is surmised that obesity resulting from BBS, which is actually a neurological condition, somehow affects the brain receptors the regulate metabolism and appetite.

In October of 2002, Myriad Genetics of Salt Lake City, Utah discovered a genetic disorder that causes obesity. A team of geneticists led by Dr. Steven Stone and Dr. Donna Shattuck isolated an obesity causing gene they named the HOB1 for Human Obesity 1. The HOB1 gene is actually a marker for certain brain functions that is somehow defective. The defect appears to inhibit the brain's ability to recognize when the body has enough fat. As a consequence of this genetic defect, those having the HOB1 gene will tend to overeat much to the point of becoming morbidly obese. The HOB1 does not appear to affect basal metabolism, but seems to relate only to energy and thermic metabolism. It is also no surprise that HOBI is linked to Type 2 Diabetes.

D. Other Causes of Obesity

It is clear that most diseases are either a cause or an effect of an imbalance in the body's normal physiological makeup. It is also clear that a change in the body's physiological makeup, whether acquired through bad habits, heredity or from a disease condition, can upset its normal metabolic actions and thus the efficiency by which it can burn calories. The result is obesity. The key to understanding the mechanism of obesity is in recognizing that it only involves two factors—what we eat and how this is burned. We must eat to survive and what we eat is burned as calories to give us energy. All that we eat which is either not burned or dispelled as waste is ultimately stored as fat. Although we can certainly control what we eat, we cannot often control how the things we eat are burned as calories. So even when we eat normally, we can still become obese and for many, many reasons.

1. Allergies

Imagine being told by your doctor that you are addicted to certain foods and that this is one of the reasons why you are obese. Many readers may recall having eaten something they like and find that despite how much of it they eat, they seem to get hungrier after having eaten it. This is actually a type of addiction that is caused by an allergic reaction to the particular food and is known as *food allergy addiction* or FAD. The mechanism of FAD is much like that of the withdrawal symptoms experienced by recovering alcoholics or drug abusers. It is an intense discomfort that actually increases the craving for the particular food allergen. When we think of an allergy, we typically view this as an adverse chemical reaction to certain substances in our environment. Usually we combat allergies by simply avoiding access to the substances that cause it. For this reason it is difficult to understand how a food allergy will actually cause us to want to consume more of the food that is causing it.

Scientists believe that contact with certain foods results in an increase in a naturally produced brain narcotic called *opioid enkephalin*. Enkephalin is a type of endorphin released by the brain to control certain behaviors; however, too much enkephalin can be likened to an addiction to heroin or opium. Consequently, when the enkephalin levels begin to drop again, the body goes into a sort of withdrawal state which is perceived as a craving for the particular food that caused the allergic reaction. This in turn leads to an insatiable appetite for the food allergen much to the point that its consumption leads to obesity.

2. Sleep Deprivation

Just as confusing as it may be to discover that food allergies can increase our appetite for the foods that cause the allergic reactions is the fact that lack of sleep can also cause obesity. Imagine that! Indeed, we have already learned that our metabolism is significantly reduced during sleep. It is also logical to assume that, when we are awake, we are certainly more active, and thus, our heart rate is faster and breathing much heavier. So, how indeed could we gain weight from lack of sleep or, more specifically, from sleep deprivation? Before answering this interesting question, it is important to recognize that numerous studies have been conducted which show that an inverse relationship exists between the number of hours of sleep and one's risk for obesity. In 2002, a study of over one million persons during a period of several years revealed that those who slept less developed a higher body mass index (BMI).

There are a number of reasons why sleep deprivation can cause obesity. First of all, lack of sleep can actually impair the body's glucose tolerance which contributes to insulin resistance and diabetes. Impaired glucose tolerance upsets the body's ability to metabolize carbohydrates which can in turn result in higher levels of fat storage. Sleep deprivation is also known to cause a decrease in the hormone *leptin*. Leptin is one of several hormones which regulate appetite. In normal patients, too much leptin will reduce appetite while too little will tend to increase appetite; however, by contrast to leptin tolerant patients, increased levels of leptin have been found in morbidly obese patients having a high resistance to the hormone. In addition to decreased levels of leptin, sleep deprivation also causes an increase in the hormone *ghrelin* which also regulates appetite. Too much ghrelin will tend to increase one's appetite. Leptin and ghrelin actually work together and are released in accordance with the body's natural clock or "human clock", a 24-hour cycle of physiological, biochemical and behavioral processes known as the *circadian rhythm*. When the circadian rhythm is disrupted by broad deviations in a person's sleep habits this results in an erratic release of these hormones that regulate appetite.

3. Stress

Although studies have shown that those under stress tend to eat more, these results suggest that, like depression and anxiety, stress is more a psychosocial cause of obesity than one of clinical origin. But as recently as 2007, it was discovered that stress can release a molecule called *neuropeptide Y* or NPY. NPY is known to actually cause an increase in both the size and number of fat cells by unlocking their receptors. Although the existence of NPY has been known since 1982, only recently has it been linked to obesity. NPY is secreted by the hypothalamus in the brain, too much of which can cause an increase in food intake corresponding to a decrease in physical activity. The decrease in physical activity derives from a type of depressed state that inhibits motivation.

An increase in the production of NPY is also now known to actually increase the proportion of energy stored as fat. Thus, the metabolism of carbohydrates is interrupted to the point that there is actually a corresponding decrease in glucose levels resulting in a temporary increase in appetite. So, in short, the reason we may eat more when were under stress follows from a real clinical basis even though stress itself is caused by our reaction to psychosocial influences.

4. Viruses and Bacteria

The way in which microorganisms can make us ill is to somehow suppress the body's immune system by destroying cells. This results in a normal metabolic reaction in which more than the usual amounts of hormones are released. As a result the body begins to retain fluids as they are needed during cell repair. But, this is the typical reaction to the effects of most viruses and bacteria. But, what if there are microorganisms which specifically interfere with normal cellular activity to increase the production of fat? Indeed, scientist have only recently discovered, for example, that the same virus which causes common respiratory and eye infections can actually alter the structure of certain stem cells, converting them into fat cells. This virus is known as the *adenovirus-36* or the AD-36 virus. Although very little is known about, AD-36, numerous studies have supported the theory that it is a definite cause of obesity in some individuals. It is believed that this virus actually modifies the structure of fat cells.

Bacteria can also cause obesity. In fact, scientists have discovered that certain microbes such as *bacteriodetes* and *firmicutes* in the stomach can promote the storage of body fat by stopping proteins from regulating its formation. These so called "bad bacteria" can also destroy the natural bacteria that help the digestion of food and thus interrupt the secretion of certain hormones, including amylase which is used to break carbohydrates down to glucose and insulin which regulates the production of glucose. It's not so much that bacteria that can cause obesity, but how bacteria in the stomach can influence digestion that should concern us. Studies have shown that obese individual have much higher levels of firmicules than individuals who are thin which suggests that these bacteria play a role at influencing the storage of fat. On the other hand, thin individuals have more bacteriodetes which suggests that these bacteria tend to influence how much food is burned as calories. In studies of animals, those without any stomach bacteria at all remained thin while those with naturally occurring stomach bacteria became overweight.

5. Therapeutic Drugs

It is clear that any drug taken into our bodies, while directly treating serious or chronic medical conditions, may also have unintended consequences on our metabolism. For example, most corticosteroids, including steroids, can cause the body to retain fluids and make us feel hungry and bloated. Corticosteroids are used primarily to treat arthritis but can increase the body's production of cortisol which can increase appetite. Neuroleptic drugs are used to treat certain psychotic conditions but can make us feel weak, lethargic and sleepy. This in turn reduces our ability to remain active thus increases our risk for obesity. Antidepressants tend to increase the body's craving for high-energy foods or those high in sugar content. High-energy foods are high in calories but have little or no nutritional value. It is interesting to note that while depression and anxiety are both precursors to obesity, the very drugs used to treat these conditions can also lead to obesity—it's like a "catch 22" or paradoxical problem. Drugs used to treat epilepsy can also contribute significantly to weight gain.

Some drugs can actually make it appear that a person is losing weight, despite the fact that he/she may be obese. Drugs such as diuretics are used to help eliminate excessive body fluids the result of which can reflect a rapid decrease in body mass. But water retention is usually only a temporary condition. In fact, some believe that the precipitous use of diuretics can help them to reduce weight and look and feel better; however, diuretics can also cause a rapid depletion in the body's electrolyte levels. Electrolytes are essential fluids whose chemical content provides the conductivity necessary to energize the body's metabolic functions like the acids in a flashlight battery. Electrolytes also provide the medium through which calories are burned. In fact, to burn calories, nutrients in the form of glucose and amino acids must be ignited just as spark plugs in an automobile ignite fuel to produce combustion. Consequently, when there is a reduction in electrolytes fewer nutrients are burned as calories are thus stored in the body as fat.

It is also true that certain medications used to treat heartburn and indigestion can cause weight gain. Drugs such as Nexium and Prevacid can actually cause weight gain in some persons because they interfere with the natural digestion of nutrients by increasing the level of sodium bicarbonate in the upper digestive tract. You may recall that sodium bicarbonate is released by the pancreas to neutralize digestive acids in chime as it passes into the duodenum. Too much sodium bicarbonate can actually reduce acid levels beyond the point that nutrients can be efficiently digested.

Drugs used to treat diabetes, such as insulin, sulfonylureas, thiazolidinedoiones can also cause weight gain. These drugs are engineered to regulate the levels of glucose in the blood stream; however, a reduction in glucose can result in hypoglycemia and induced hunger. This in turn can result in weight gain. Studies have shown, in fact, that these drugs and result in an average weight gain of 5.1 kilograms over several weeks of use.

6. Aging

If we consume the exact same quantity of foods in terms of their caloric content throughout our lives, our activity levels held constant, as we get older we will inevitably begin to gain weight. The reason for this that the body's metabolic rates eventually become less efficient, just as our muscles weaken and our bones become more brittle—all consequences of aging. Age is actually a double-edge sword in favor of the development of an obese state. In addition to having a physiologically reduced metabolic rate, older people tend to be less active. Reduced activity is usually not a function of choice. The aging process actually begins to weaken us. This results primarily from a reduction in sex hormones through the menopausal state in both males and females. A reduction in these hormones can result in weight gain and a redistribution of fat.

Studies have shown that the levels of testosterone in the testes of males and ovaries of females are significantly diminished with age, even before menopause. Testosterone is the principal hormone that regulates the body's *anabolic effects*. The anabolic effects refer to the growth of muscle mass and increased bone density. Clearly, when there is a reduction in the levels of testosterone the anabolic effects will begin to diminish as well. The anabolic effects begin at about age 9 and will peak through puberty. It levels off at about age 25 and then, at about age 30, begins slowly declining. After age 50 the anabolic effects are scarcely involved in body metabolism and thus, activity levels begin to fall off rapidly. Muscle mass diminishes and muscles begin to weaken. Bone mass also diminishes and may change its structure. As a result of this significant decrease in the anabolic effects, bones become more brittle and susceptible to injury.

People begin to gain weight as they age especially if they do not modify their eating habits. This is true of many athletes whose vigorous life styles suddenly end upon early retirement from whatever sports activity they may have been involved. It is extremely difficult to jump immediately from a diet of 5,000 calories per day to one of less than 2,500 per day and thus, many athletes spend years in adjustment. Some become obese and remain that way throughout the remainder of their lives. Others tend to struggle with weight gain for many years before settling into their less active life. Retirement is actually considered a functional cause of obesity simply because of the immediate change in lifestyle that results. Even though retired individuals often now have more time to be active, especially if their careers imposed a sedentary life style, they usually tend to become more sedentary regardless. Most retired persons tend to engage in leisurely, non-stress-inducing activities. They also tend to travel more and will thus eat out at restaurants where prepared foods are not always healthy. Retired persons also develop more illnesses more frequently and thus will be prescribed drugs which may adversely affect metabolism.

E. Chapter Summary

The popular belief is that obesity is caused by lack of exercise and over-eating. While this is true to some extent, obesity is in fact the result of multiple predisposing factors many of which are not at all our fault or even under our immediate control. It is indeed true that if we eat more than our body's can effectively metabolize, unless we somehow burn the calories that result, we will gain weight. The key phrase here is "effectively metabolize". Because metabolism requires a delicate balance of chemicals that regulate how we burn calories for energy, any deficiency in the complex processing plant that energizes the body can result in weight gain despite any disciplined regimen of diet and exercise. In general, there are three major areas of influence upon metabolism—psychosocial, medical condition (including injury and disease) and heredity.

The psychosocial effects upon metabolism consist of those factors that result from our behavior, attitudes and perceptions. These include our lifestyles, personality type, the influence of alcohol, drug abuse and smoking, career profiles, how we deal with depression and anxiety and, of course, what and how we eat. Our lifestyles will place us into one of three general categories of behavior: active-aggressive, passive-aggressive or passive-sedentary. Those who are active-aggressive would be least likely to become obese while those who are passive-sedentary would be most likely to become obese. Our personality profiles put most of us on a range from Type A or aggressive to Type B or relaxed with the latter being more likely than the former to become obese. The way we manage stress through alcohol and drug abuse can have a significant influence upon whether or not we will become obese and, while smoking, may increase our metabolism, it can also increase appetite. Depression and anxiety can influence the balance of hormones that regulate appetite. Obesity can also result from eating just one large meal a day and this, just before going to bed at night, rather than several small meals at regular intervals during the day.

There are numerous medical conditions and disease states that can influence the hormone balance of our bodies. Hypothyroidism can cause weight gain from a change in the hormones that regulate appetite. Cushing's disease results from a high concentration of cortisol, a natural steroid that upsets the body's blood sugar levels leading to obesity. Polycystic Ovary Disease results in high levels of the hormone androgen in females which can lead to obesity. Metabolic syndrome is a collection of medical conditions that results in a reduction in the body's metabolic rate also leading to obesity.

Obesity can also be inherited. Although we can easily be influenced by the behavior of obese parents, this is something within our control; however, certain genetic markers called DNA (deoxyribonucleic acid) passed onto us from our obese parents can actually lead us into a life of obesity despite what we do to prevent it. Scientist have isolated a so called "fat gene" which may have evolved over many years from early tribal cultures that would store large amounts of fat, like bears preparing for hibernation and/or survival during periods of famine. It has also been proven that certain psychosocial behaviors can be passed to offspring, including personality and a tendency to become alcoholics, smokers and drug abusers.

Other causes of obesity include allergies, sleep deprivation, stress, use of therapeutic drugs and the aging process. Allergic reactions to certain foods can act much like a drug or alcohol withdrawal symptom. Instead of avoiding foods containing the allergen, we instead become addicted and thus develop an intense a craving and voracious appetite for such foods. Stress increases the release and presence of cortisol resulting in an increase in blood sugar levels. This can cause diabetes as well as obesity. The use of therapeutic drugs tends to upset the delicate balance of our metabolism and result eventually in obesity. One of the many effects of aging is a diminished metabolism as well as a reduction in activity resulting from general weakening of bones and muscles. Aging is also consistent with a reduction in the sex hormones that give us the drive and motivation to be physically active.

Key Points:

1. Obesity is caused, for various reasons, by the body's inability to metabolize all that we consume
2. Obesity can be caused by the way we are influenced by factors in our environment such as lifestyle, personality traits, career choice, etc
3. Alcoholism and drug abuse are associated with obesity
4. Obesity can result from certain medical conditions such as hypothyroidism, Cushing's Disease and Metabolic Syndrome
5. Allergies, viruses and bacteria can cause obesity
6. Obesity can be caused by certain drugs that we use
7. Obesity can be inherited genetically or through behavioral influences
8. Stress, depression and anxiety can lead to obesity
9. Risk of obesity increases with age

Chapter 4--*Dangers of Obesity*

Many persons who become obese eventually develop a comfort level with their condition. Some may venture into denial and thus hang out, so to speak, with other obese individuals to help support their adopted behavior. Some individuals may even sustain the belief that being obese as quite normal and acceptable. But, on the contrary, obesity is an invitation to a litany of health problems, many of which can be fatal. It's not enough that being obese is culturally unacceptable in modern society. Obese individuals often suffer from serious and chronic health conditions. They can also succumb to severe depression and anxiety that may result from being a so called "freak" and socially outcast. Depression and anxiety are causally linked to many serious health conditions, including hypertension and heart disease. Obesity is also a formidable survivor in that this condition itself can lead to a sluggish and sedentary life style that makes matters even worse.

It is important to recognize that overweight or obese individuals store more fat than the body needs to survive. This excess fat has weight that makes it seem much like carrying a suitcase around all day, every day. Overweight persons tend to get tired more easily and thus engage in less activity. While many deal with the problem through diet and exercise, drug therapy and/or surgery, others take drastic and dangerous measures to control their weight, including smoking, long periods of fasting and, at the extreme end, binge eating and purging. These activities all can become predispositions to serious, often fatal health conditions.

A. Direct Medical Risks Associated with Diabetes

Whether or not it is derived from sheer lifestyle or matters out of our immediate control, obesity is a problem which must be managed for the sake of our own health. As a long-term condition, obesity eventually takes its toll on the body and begins to rare its ugly head in unexpected and deleterious ways. In many ways, obesity is like smoking or alcohol abuse. At some point it will have an effect upon our health. Indeed, if we continue to drive a car without ever changing the oil, the latter will begin to break down into a useless substance and result in irreparable damage to the car's engine. In similar fashion, we must now and then clean out the drain pipe of an air conditioner or drain the water from the reservoir of a water heater. If not, sediments will accumulate to the point that serious harm can result to the equipment.

The human body can withstand a great many things. It is durable and resilient, yet delicate and sensitive. Being overweight or obese is not itself a serious problem, as long as the body is given a means to recover from this condition. Many individuals become overweight or perhaps obese for short periods, but make the conscientious decision to manage the problem.

Once the overweight condition is resolved, so too are the underlying health risks. But, long-term, unresolved obesity may eventually give in to serious medical conditions such as diabetes, heart disease, hypertension, respiratory dysfunction, gall bladder disease and many others.

1. Insulin Resistance and Diabetes

In **Chapter 2**, you may recall from our discussion of the digestive system, how foods are reduced to a state that is easily absorbed into the blood stream. Foods are broken down by chemicals called hormones which are secreted or released by various glands along the alimentary canal (the path that food takes from the mouth to the rectum). One of the most important digestive glands is the pancreas. You may recall that this gland releases several hormones and chemicals during the digestive process, among these being insulin. Insulin is very important in the metabolism of glucose. Recall that carbohydrates are converted to glucose by an enzyme called amylase which is secreted first in the mouth by the salivary glands and then again in the duodenum by the pancreas. The pancreas not only secretes digestive enzymes to help break food down to a substance more readily absorbable into the blood stream, but also produces insulin as a means of controlling an over production of glucose.

Insulin is produced by the beta cells in that part of the pancreas known as the *Islet of Langerhans*, which was discovered in 1869 by anatomical pathologist, Paul Langerhans. The name insulin was derived coincidentally from the Latin word, *insula* which is means "island". The purpose of insulin is to gather glucose from the blood and to store it in liver and muscle as *glycogen*. Glycogen is held in storage accordingly until it is needed by the body for energy during periods of fasting or starvation when is converted back again to glucose. Without insulin, too much glucose will be produced thus causing a rise in blood sugar levels. Too much sugar in the blood can result in a condition known as hyperglycemia. In some individuals, hyperglycemia occurs sometimes, but only temporarily when, insulin levels either decline or become deficient. This can occur, for example, if vigorous exercise is preceded by the ingestion of candy or a meal high in sugar content. A consistent or chronic increase in blood-sugar levels resulting from a decline in the levels of insulin or from insulin resistance can be a precursor to more serious complications the most notable of which is called Type 2 Diabetes. Hyperglycemia can also cause a serious complication known as ketaoacidosis from an over-production of ketones which can be fatal. Ketoacidosis occurs frequently among diabetics.

a. Insulin Resistance

The most common cause of hyperglycemia is insulin resistance. In fact, approximately one out of every three persons will develop some degree of insulin resistance, a condition which is characterized by the body's inability to properly utilize insulin. Although insulin resistance can be inherited, it is also a consequence of obesity, stress, infection, steroid use and certain drugs. It may also result from a sedentary life style, aging, especially for those over 40 years old, and/or those who are glucose intolerant. It occurs most commonly in Latinos, Asian-Americans, African-Americans and Pacific Islanders. Among the most remarkable consequences of insulin resistance is that the rise in blood sugar resulting from this condition can increase appetite, so that while the condition can be a consequence of obesity, it can also result in obesity—hence, another "catch 22".

Insulin resistance is really not an under-production of insulin. In fact, those who have it often produce too much insulin; but, it simply cannot efficiently regulate glucose levels. What happens is that, as the glucose levels rise, the pancreas responds naturally by producing more and more insulin to overcompensate. Scientists believe that the body's ability to process insulin at the cellular level becomes somehow deficient as a result of obesity, aging or an abnormal accumulation of triglycerides and other factors as discussed above. A deficiency in the value of insulin complicates matters in that many patients with hyperglycemia cannot be treated simply by an injection of insulin to regulate glucose. Instead, they must restrict their diets by reducing carbohydrate and sugar intake in order to manage glucose levels accordingly.

b. Type 2 Diabetes

The most serious complication of insulin resistance is Type 2 Diabetes resulting from consistently high levels of glucose in the blood over a period of many years. This occurs either because insulin has become ineffective itself at regulating glucose levels or the body's cell structure has become ineffective at processing insulin. As a result, the levels of glucose begin to rise and accumulate in the blood stream causing serious collateral health problems. Individuals with Type 2 Diabetes will usually experience frequent bouts of hyperglycemia.

Numerous studies have been conducted which support the theory that obesity can lead to Type 2 Diabetes. This theory follows from a direct correlation between this disease and individuals who are obese or consistently overweight, especially in the abdominal area. Although anyone can acquire the disease, it is most prevalent among those having an abnormally high body mass index (BMI). More than 2.8% of world's population now consists of persons with Type 2 Diabetes. In fact, Type 2 Diabetes is now the sixth leading cause of death in the United States. Death usually results from long-term complications or untreated conditions that can result from Type 2 Diabetes. The collateral problems caused by Type 2 Diabetes include nerve damage, hypertension or high blood pressure, heart disease, kidney disease, stroke and blindness. Those with Type 2 Diabetes are especially deficient in their ability to heal from injuries to the extremities such as feet and hands. In many instances, they may develop gangrene and thus require amputation. Type 2 Diabetics are also more likely to acquire neoplasms (cancer) of the digestive tract, including colon cancer, pancreatic cancer, esophageal and stomach cancer.

c. Monitoring Blood Sugar Levels

It is very important to recognize the early symptoms of diabetes. Persons with frequent episodes of hyperglycemia at any age will likely develop Type 2 Diabetes. Hyperglycemia resulting from insulin resistance is easily monitored by continually measuring blood sugar levels and managing these levels accordingly. Blood sugar is easily measured using home testing kits available from most drug stores or pharmacies. In fact, many doctors recommend that everyone begin testing blood sugar levels regularly after age 45 and everyone who suffers from occasional hyperglycemia should test at any age. Normal blood sugar levels will fall within a range from 70 mg/dl to 100 mg/dl. The usage "mg/dl" means the quantity of glucose in milligrams per deciliter of blood. Blood sugar levels will generally be at their lowest level in the mornings after waking, but will rise significantly after a meal.

Although testing for blood sugar levels is highly recommended for those with Type 2 Diabetes, there is really no clear cut rule on the frequency at which such testing should be done. For those who experience occasional bouts of hyperglycemia, random testing levels if done at least once each day at different times may be acceptable, but for those with chronic hyperglycemia and those with Type 2 Diabetes, blood sugar monitoring should be conducted according to a specific regimentation at least once each day. A popular testing regimen for those who may be at risk for acquiring Type 2 Diabetes is referred to as a fasting glucose test or, more specifically, *fasting plasma glucose* (FPG). This test is done after about 8 hours without eating in order to establish whether or not the blood sugar levels will decline to their normal levels long after a meal. If the results of this test reveal blood sugar levels anywhere between 100 mg/dl and 125 mg/dl this is considered as impaired fasting glucose and a precursor to Type 2 Diabetes. A diagnosis of Type 2 Diabetes is determined for any levels above 126 mg/dl with this test.

The reason that the FPG test is important is that blood sugar levels will increase naturally immediately after a meal, sometimes to as high as 180 mg/dl. As the food is being digested, the pancreas is expected to produce insulin immediately to begin regulating blood sugar levels until the meal is fully digested. This process takes about four hours, so at the end of eight hours, one would expect the blood sugar levels to fall well below 100 mg/dl. If not, then it is likely that the tested individual is insulin resistant and probably a Type 2 Diabetic. In this case, exercise, and a strict diet high in protein and low in carbohydrates and sugar is recommended. Exercise is especially important. Remember that glucose is burned in the form of calories to provide energy. Consequently, when the glucose levels in the blood are high, it is important to somehow increase the body's need for energy either by becoming more active or by engaging in some form of exercise. In some cases, especially for insulin resistant patients and those who are unable to exercise, medication may be required to regulate blood sugar levels. There are literally dozens of drugs used to manage insulin resistance and are prescribed according to the special circumstances of each respective patient.

2. Cancer

Obesity has been linked to many types of cancer most notably those that involve the digestive system. These include esophageal and stomach cancer, pancreatic cancer and colorectal cancer. Although scientists are not clear on why obesity is linked to cancer, studies have shown a higher incidence of these types of cancer in overweight and obese individuals than in those with normal body mass. The most notable link between obesity and cancer is insulin resistance. It is believed that insulin resistance, which causes the pancreas to over produce insulin, may stimulate cell proliferation which can trigger the onset of neoplasms. A neoplasm, commonly known as cancer, is precisely what its Latin name suggests "neo" for new and "plasm" for cell. These new cells can grow uncontrollably, consuming the body's natural resources to the point of actually killing us.

Then notion of cell proliferation as being the precursor of cancer in obese individuals derives from another, but highly controversial theory that the body's reaction to increased body mass is to "fill-in" the gap in order to balance the differential between fat and other body tissue. This theory suggests that we can actually continue to grow, but not necessarily in accordance with the patterns of our DNA. The theory does not explain why people of normal weight can also acquire cancer. As a general perspective, despite what may be the underlying cause, it is clear from statistical studies that obese individuals have a 30% to 40% greater likelihood of developing certain cancers than individuals of normal weight.

3. Hypertension and Stroke

When the heart beats, it contracts and expands. When it contracts, it pumps or pushes blood into the circulatory system causing an increase in the pressure against the walls of the blood vessels (veins and arteries). This is called the *systolic rhythm* or systolic pressure. When the heart expands, it draws blood into itself thus causing a reduction in pressure. This is called the *diastolic rhythm* or diastolic pressure. Pressure against the walls of the blood vessels is measured using a standardized scale for the weight of one atmosphere per millimeter of mercury or mm/Hg. Without actually describing this measure, an example can be given by what happens when you squeeze a balloon filled with water. If you let the balloon dangle undisturbed, this would be the diastolic pressure. When you squeeze the balloon, this applies force against the inside. If you squeeze too hard, the balloon could burst.

The normal amount of pressure applied to the walls of the blood vessels using the standard scale is 120 mm/Hg over 80 mm/Hg or 120/80, or in the terms introduced above, systolic over diastolic pressure. This means that when the heart contracts it will increase the pressure against the walls of the blood vessels up to 120 mm/hg and when the heart expands, this will drop the pressure against the wall of the vessels down to about 80 mm/Hg. This is normal pressure when the body is at rest. When engaged in strenuous activity or when under stress, the pressure will rise, but only temporarily; however, when the pressure rises and stays there for extended periods, even at rest, this is a condition known a *hypertension*, more commonly referred to as high blood pressure. A sustained systolic pressure greater than 150 mm/Hg, coupled with a diastolic pressure greater than 90 mm/Hg at rest is considered too high.

Hypertension is the leading cause of stroke and heart disease. Hypertension can also cause aneurisms which are weakened areas of the arterial walls that can expand and burst during the systolic cycle of the heart. Although the causes of hypertension are not clearly understand, studies have shown that it exists almost invariably in individuals who are overweight or obese. In fact, more than 70% of obese individuals will develop hypertension. Hypertension is especially prevalent among individuals having abdominal adiposity or the so called "beer belly". The cause of hypertension among obese individuals is believed to be attributed to changes in the neuroendocrine mechanism.

The neuroendocrine system regulates a complex plant known as the renin-angiotensin-aldosterone system which regulates the volume of blood in the body as well as how the body retains and dispels fluids. It also controls the sympathetic nervous system and regulates the amount of sodium or salt that is retained by the body. When the body begins to accumulate fat, this results in the accumulation of sodium and corresponding retention of fluids. This in turn results in an increase in blood volume. The way this works is sort of like increasing the amount of water flow into a hose that is sealed at the other end. As more water is pushed into the hose, this will eventually cause its walls to expand. As this condition continues over time, the hose will begin to weaken at various points and rupture. This is precisely what happens with a stroke caused by cerebral hemorrhage, bleeding into the brain from a ruptured blood vessel.

4. Kidney Disease

Among the most important organs is the body are the kidneys. These are bean shaped organs located in the area of the lower back which separate waste products such as urea, mineral salts and toxins from the blood. These wastes are gathered and filtered by the kidneys then dumped into a reservoir called the bladder from which they are released by us as urine.

Although the kidneys function largely to regulate and eliminate waste, they also act to retain water, sodium and electrolytes all of which together act like acids in a flashlight battery to provide a medium of electrical energy.

Scientists believe that obesity causes an increase in the re-absorption of renal sodium. This can result in a decrease in urine output and thus an increase in fluid retention. Fluid retention can cause edema or swelling of the extremities (arms and legs) and also an increase in blood pressure. High blood pressure can also cause serious kidney damage and thus reduce the efficiency by which body fluids are dispelled as waste.

5. Cardiovascular Disease

Aside from stroke caused by hypertension, probably the most serious complication of obesity is cardiovascular disease which itself can be caused most notably by hypertension. Since we now know that hypertension can result from being obese, it follows that cardiovascular disease is also at least indirectly a consequence of obesity. Cardiovascular disease includes a collection of serious medical conditions such as coronary artery disease, congestive heart disease, certain vascular conditions such as aneurisms, venous insufficiency, athroma and arteriosclerosis and cardiac arrhythmias.

Although hypertension is a major predisposition to cardiovascular disease there are other, more insidious causes. The way in which the heart circulates blood throughout the body is a process known as *hemodynamics*. Hemodynamics refers the amount of output required by the heart to maintain the body's necessary oxygen needs, especially during high activity levels. The more active the body becomes the greater will be its hemodynamic rate. But, the hemodynamic rate can also increase for other reasons. Among these is an increase in the circulation of adipose tissue in the blood that can gradually and slowly accumulate and congeal sort of like sediment in a water pipe, thus causing serious impairment of the circulatory system. Constriction of the circulatory system in this way causes the heart to work much harder thus increasing its hemodynamic rate.

Hemodynamic heart activity can also increase as a result of the increased metabolic demand that is induced by excessive body weight. Overweight individuals carry more weight than normal individuals and thus require more energy to handle this excess baggage. Obviously, it requires more strength to lift 100 pounds than it does to lift 10 pounds. In response to this higher demand for energy, the heart will work harder even when the body is at rest. Because the heart is more active at rest among obese individuals this can also inhibit sleep, thus making matters even worsen.

Obesity can also result in certain vascular diseases. The term vascular refers to anything related to blood. The veins, arteries, and capillaries are all part of the vascular system. Among the more common vascular conditions resulting from obesity is venous insufficiency resulting in pedal edema. The latter condition can cause pooling of blood and clotting in the lower extremities. This can cause edema or swelling and severe pain in the lower legs. Obesity has also been associated with an increased risk of pulmonary emboli in women. A pulmonary embolism is a blood clot in the lungs which can be caused by venous insufficiency, deep vein thrombosis (phlebitis) and increased hemodynamic heart rate. Because pulmonary emboli can cause sudden death, it is an extremely serious consequence of obesity.

6. Gallbladder Disease

The gallbladder is a very small organ located just under the lower liver. Its primary function is to store and concentrate bile which is produced in the liver to aid in the digestive process. When it is needed, the gallbladder releases bile into the duodenum to digest fat. Under certain conditions, especially among overweight or obese individuals, a decrease in natural bile salts known as *bilirubin* can result in the accumulation of cholesterol. This accumulation can result in bile being trapped in the gallbladder. As cholesterol continues to accumulate in the gallbladder this substance can harden to form stones whose eventual release into the common bile duct can cause severe pain. The stones formed by hardened cholesterol are commonly referred to as "gall stones". When gall stones increase in size and quantity they can also irritate the inner lining of the gallbladder resulting in a condition known as cholecystitis or inflammation of the gallbladder.

In Western culture, the gallbladder is, in many ways, much like the appendix and not always needed; however, an increase in the consumption of foods high in fat content can increase gallbladder activity. It is important to understand that the gallbladder's primary function is to digest fat, so the less fat we consume the less active will be the gallbladder. In fact, during episodes of severe pain resulting from the release of gallstone into the common bile duct, the immediate elimination of fat, coupled with certain medications to help dissolve gall stones can provide relief. Sometimes, however, it is necessary to remove the gallbladder altogether through a very simple procedure known as a cholecystectomy. Since removal of the gallbladder will significantly reduce the efficiency by which fat is digested and metabolized those without this organ must eliminate fat in their diets almost completely or take medications to assist in the digestion of fat.

Scientists are not clear why bilirubin (bile salt) levels will decrease in overweight individuals. Some believe it to be hormonal but others maintain that the high levels of cholesterol from the intake of fat can envelop bile salts in the gallbladder thus making the organ less effective at releasing bile. What happens is that the cholesterol sort of dams up the gallbladder, preventing bile produced in the liver from being injected into it and also from being released to digest fat.

7. Osteoarthritis

The area at which one bone joins another as for example the bones of the lower leg with that of the upper leg is called a joint. In the lower leg are the fibula and tibia, both of which are connected at the knee joint to the upper leg bone which is called the femur. If the bones simply come together at the joint without some type of lubricate, they will rub against each other, eventually wearing out and, of course, causing severe pain in the process. For this reason, a soft, flexible, bone-like material called *cartilage* lies between these bones at the joint. Cartilage not only helps to cushion the joint but also provides a sort of adhesive connection point, thus preventing the bones from slipping off of each other.

In overweight and obese individuals more pressure applied to the joints from excessive weight, especially at the knees and hips will cause these joints to eventually wear resulting in a condition known as *osteoarthritis* or inflammation of the joints. Osteoarthritis can also occur among individuals of normal weight who run or jog frequently, but a causal relationship is not clear considering that many who jog do not develop osteoarthritis. Osteoarthritis is also a degenerative disease having no specific etiology or cause other than it is among the consequences of aging. One thing that is very clear about osteoarthritis is that there is a statistically higher prevalence of this condition among those who are obese and its prevalence is directly proportional to a person's weight.

8. Sleep Apnea

Because overweight and obese individuals tend to have a higher hemodynamic rate, including increased respiration and heart activity, this tends to make it difficult for them to experience normal sleep. More importantly, however, is that obesity can cause serious respiratory complications because obese individuals have an increased demand for blood oxygenation. In fact, obesity is a classic cause of a condition known as *alveolar hypoventilation* or more specifically, *obesity hypoventilation syndrome (OBS)*. Those with OBS will also develop what is called the "pickwickian" syndrome which is also known as sleep apnea. Sleep apnea is a serious health condition which results when breathing stops or pauses frequently during sleep.

With normal breathing, the lungs expand to draw in oxygen and contract to release carbon dioxide. During this process, there are levels of both oxygen and carbon dioxide in the blood stream. These are known as blood gases. During sleep, when breathing is interrupted, this results in less oxygen being absorbed into the blood stream. It also results in an increase in the levels of carbon dioxide in the blood stream. Too much carbon dioxide in the blood stream results in a condition known as *hypercapnia* which can cause severe headaches, confusion and lithargy (fatigue). Hypercapnia can also lead to increased cardiac output and hypertension leading to cardiac arrest. Too little oxygen in the blood stream can lead to *hypoxemia* which causes a temporary condition known as *hypoxia*. Hypoxia resulting in a lack of sufficient oxygen to the brain can cause vertigo (dizziness) and unconsciousness.

B. Collateral Medical Risks Associated with Obesity

It's not enough that obesity comes with serious and often deadly medical risks, but it also can alter behavior to the point that drastic measures are undertaken to counteract the condition. More often than not, individuals who begin to experience weight gain will overcompensate in ways which are not only creative but potentially harmful. For example, many alcoholics will simply stop eating to avoid gaining weight from the consumption of alcohol. This means essentially that alcohol becomes their only source of nutrition. Consequently, many of the essential vitamins and minerals obtained through normal dieting are then eliminated. As a result, the body develops a condition known as *wasting syndrome* in which the muscle and bones begin to lose mass.

The self-consciousness among overweight or obese individuals tend to engage in harmful practices such as long-term starvation and aggressive exercise. Starvation can lead to severe malnutrition and aggressive exercise to serious injury. In both such instances, the risk of cardiac arrest is significantly increased.

1. Anorexia (Anorexia Nervosa)

In some individuals, especially those with low self-esteem and an obsessive fear of gaining weight, a behavioral disorder can result in which anything and everything is done to avoid gaining weight. This can lead to a serious medical condition known as *anorexia nervosa*, a chronic eating disorder which can be fatal if not treated Anorexic (or anorectic) individuals maintain a much lower than normal body weight to overcompensate for their fear of becoming obese. These individuals believe that, by so doing, their likelihood of becoming obese is significantly reduced. Many individuals at one time or another have adopted behavior similar to those who are anorexic, but only to overcompensate temporarily for an overweight condition. Anorexia, on the other hand, is a long-term behavioral disorder that comes with often more serious clinical side effects than obesity itself.

Anorexic individuals are easily recognized by the various overt symptoms that manifest themselves with this condition. In addition to being conspicuously skinny or underweight, those with anorexia also suffer from a condition known as *lanugo* which is characterized by an abnormal increase in facial and body hair. Anorexia also causes severe dental and orthodontic issues including cavities, tooth loss and gum disease or gingivitis, most probably from a lack of calcium and other essential minerals. Anorexia can lead to swollen joints and severe abdominal distention or bloated abdomen. In many ways, alcoholics and those suffering from anorexia have symptoms in common. Most anorexics can be identified by their puffy cheeks which results from the enlargement of the salivary glands. Because those with anorexia have virtually no body fat, they will become intolerant of the cold.

Anorexia is also characterized by bazaar deviations in behavior. Anorexic individuals tend to have an obsession with food, recipes, calorie content and cooking and may even cook complex and elaborate meals for everyone else but themselves. They also avoid eating around others and will tend to cut their foods into tiny portions and eat very slowly. Moreover, anorexic individual will also engage in very strenuous exercise and quite to the point of endangering their health. Even though they are clearly underweight, they will perceive themselves as being overweight nevertheless and will constantly seek verbal affirmation. Anorexic individuals also tend become antisocial, always wear loose-fitting clothes and suffer chronically from depression and anxiety.

Other conditions which result from anorexia include but are not necessarily limited to those in **Table X** below.

Table X : Clinical Manifestations of Anorexia	
Condition or Disease	**Characteristics**
Acne	Excessive distribution of pusculated lesions or pimples on the skin
Seborrheic Dermatitis	Greasy, scaly and flaky skin
Hyperpigmentation	Darkening of the skin
Pellagra	Amino acid deficiency from lack of protein and the vitamin niacin
Paroanychia	Inflammation of the nail fold
Constipation	Obstruction of bowel movement
Diarrhea	Frequent and watery stool

Table X : Clinical Manifestations of Anorexia	
Condition or Disease	**Characteristics**
Osteoporosis	Reduced bone mineral density
Cardiac Arrest	Heart attack or sudden death of the heart
Hyponatremia	Dangerous loss of sodium in the body
Brain Atrophy	Loss of brain tissue resulting in seizure disorder
Amenorrhea	Absence of menstrual cycle in woman of reproductive age
Electrolyte Deficiency	Dehydration

Anorexia is much more common in women than men, primarily because of the social and cultural pressures that prevail upon how women should appear. This is especially true among those in the public eye such as celebrities and politicians. In fact, anorexia gained widespread attention in 1983 following the sudden death from this disease of singer-songwriter and percussionist Karen Carpenter. The news of Carpenter's death from anorexia soon gave in to a media storm which uncovered many other cases mostly involving female celebrities. Among these were Sandra Dee, Sally Field, Jane Fonda, Mariel Hemingway, Kate Beckinsale, Paula Abdul, Marie Osmond, Britney Spears, Audrey Hepburn, Kate Winslet, Oprah Winfrey and Diana, Princess of Wales. Anorexia also found its way into the ranks of many popular male celebrities such as Elvis Presley, Elton John, Richard Simmons and Dennis Quaid.

2. Bulimia (Bulimia Nervosa)

With anorexia, eating is actually a clinical repulsion. Anorexics tend to avoid eating until they are so hungry that they simply have no choice but to eat something. When they do eat it is very little and very infrequent. A psychotic condition that is closely related to anorexia is one in which eating becomes an obsession, but not to the detriment of one's weight. Instead of resisting food to avoid gaining weight, this obsession involves long periods of fasting coupled intermittently with short bouts of binge or voracious eating. Those having this condition avoid gaining weight by eating excessive amounts of food and then purging it by compensatory behavior or self-induced vomiting. This condition is known as *bulimia nervosa* or bulimia for short. Bulimia is a very serious condition in that this behavior places an extreme amount of metabolic stress upon the body.

The behavior of bulimic individuals is precarious at best. Unlike anorexic individuals, those suffering from bulimia will appear quite normal and healthy; however, the long-term consequences of their behavior are almost always fatal, ending usually in severe cardiac stress and heart attack. With most bulimic individuals, they may eat small meals on a daily basis, but occasionally will undertake to devour large quantities of food to appease their voracious appetites, sometimes as much as 10,000 calories per day. Then, overcome with feelings of guilt and remorse, will immediately run to the bathroom and induce vomiting. Aside from the heightened metabolic rate induced by voracious and rapid intake of food, its sudden release from vomiting confuses the body's hemodynamic rate which can induce heart attack. Even if the bulimic individual survives it, vomiting almost invariably results in an immediate and dangerous loss of electrolytes. It can also damage the lining of the stomach, the esophagus and the throat. In some cases, self-induced vomiting can cause auto-aspiration, a condition in which the vomit can inadvertently pass into the trachea and choke the victim.

Victims of bulimia will also take large amounts of laxatives and exercise vigorously between meals. Both such extremes further exacerbate the stress bulimia places upon the cardiovascular system. Because voracious short-term binges tend to also rapidly expand the stomach lining, bulimic individuals will feel hungrier than a normal individual while in a state of fasting. For this reason, many recovering bulimics tend to become obese anyway. In some cases victims of bulimia have actually eaten to the point that their stomachs have ruptured. As a result, the acidic contents of their stomachs infiltrate into the peritoneum causing severe pain and possible death.

Because large amounts of foods are consumed during a very short period with this disease, digestive hormones and chemicals, including the acids of the stomach begin rapidly over-producing. When the stomach is then immediately purged from self-induced vomiting, these acids remain for longer than normal periods. This causes severe gastric distress, acid reflux, indigestion and ulcers. Another little known consequence of bulimia is hiatus hernia (pl., hiatal hernias). A hiatus hernia results when the point at which the esophagus attaches to the stomach moves up, along with part of the stomach, above the diaphragm. The diaphragm separates the lungs and heart from the lower abdomen and the stomach rests just below and against it. When back pressure builds from frequent bouts of self-induced vomiting, this can pull part of the stomach upward and into the chest. The result is chronic acid reflux, digestive discomfort and, in extreme case, constriction and tissue destruction of the stomach lining.

3. Malnutrition

An obvious consequence of defensive behavior against the onset of obesity is the potential lack of proper nutrition that results. Anorexic individuals are particularly susceptible to vitamin and mineral deficiency. Many anorexics will consume large quantities of vitamin and mineral supplements to offset the nutritional deficiencies that result from their behavior. But, vitamins in particular can actually increase one's appetite. Faced with this complication, many anorexics will avoid taking vitamins and thus further exacerbate their condition.

Lack of the proper intake of nutrients, including vitamins and minerals, results in a potentially serious condition known as malnutrition. Malnutrition results not only from anorexic behavior, but also from improper dieting and also from bulimia. Malnutrition can result from taking in too much of a particular vitamin, especially if this is a fat-soluble vitamin. For example, too much Vitamin D can result in a condition known as hypervitaminosis D. On the other hand, too little of this vitamin can cause Rickets. Other conditions such as Scurvy from lack of vitamin C and Beri Beri from lack of vitamin B can also result from malnutrition. Scurvy can cause severe diarrhea, dehydration and dangerous loss of electrolytes. Beri Beri can result in permanent damage to the nervous, gastrointestinal, cardiovascular and muscular systems. Malnutrition can also result in iodine deficiency which can cause variety of mental disorders.

Malnutrition can also result from eating normal amounts of the wrong food. For example, the excess consumption of lean meat, coupled with a lack of sufficient carbohydrates and fats can result in a condition known as "Rabbit Starvation", or more specifically, protein poisoning. This behavior can result in serious medical complications, including diarrhea, low blood pressure and heart rate. It can also result in headaches, fatigue and an intense craving for certain foods, especially those containing carbohydrates and fat. The phrase "Rabbit Starvation" derived from conditions observed among forest Indian tribes of North America who often fed almost exclusively on Rabbits. Unlike the meat of beaver, moose, fish and similar such game which is high in concentrated fat, rabbit meat is the leanest in North America

4. Ketosis

One of the many ways in which individuals combat obesity is by fasting or going long periods without eating anything at all. During this fasting stage, the body initially goes into starvation mode in order to preserve energy. But, after a certain period, the fat that is stored in the body is then called upon and converted to energy. This conversion process results in the accumulation of a sort of digestive acid or waste product known as *ketones*. With normal metabolism, energy is derived from glucose converted from carbohydrates; but, any excess amount of glucose is converted and stored in the body as fat. When fat is converted to energy, ketones are used as fuel instead of glucose.

When fasting for very long periods, as is often the case with those suffering from anorexia, this can result in an over accumulation of ketones in the body. Too much of this acid causes a condition known as ketosis. Ketosis can make you feel tired, weak and thirsty. It can also cause headaches and vomiting. Those who suffer from ketosis can also develop halitosis or malodorous breath. Although ketosis can occur among those who fast for long periods, it is also prevalent in persons on a diet low in carbohydrates. With a low-carbohydrate diet, less glucose is available for energy, so the body reacts by converting fat to ketones.

5. Inactivity

One of the problems with obesity is that this condition tends to increase the amount of energy required by the body even at rest. In many ways, obese individuals feel as though they have been walking, biking or jogging all day because of how their condition can task their bodies. Being obesity makes a person feel sluggish, lethargic and unwieldy. After all, obese individuals are carrying considerably more weight than was naturally intended by the body. As a consequence of the sluggishness derived from their condition, obese individuals tend to adopt a less active and more sedentary lifestyle. In short, they become so called "couch potatoes", a condition that makes matters even worse.

Unlike the highly defensive measures against obesity such as anorexia and bulimia, lack of physical activity is a complete resignation from the condition itself. Overweight and obese individuals who engage in a sedentary lifestyle are actually in a psychotic state of denial and thus have accepted and adopted their condition as being normal. These individuals tend to avoid making appearances in public. If they do engage in social interaction it is usually done so with other obese individuals. This behavior can even evolve to the point that the obese individuals will rail upon those who are thin and active and often tell them that they look sickly, unhealthy or anorexic. Such individuals may also cajole others to eat more. They will buy clothes that make them look thinner or those that are baggy in an attempt to hide their condition.

Inactivity among overweight and obese individuals can eventually lead to morbid obesity which is potentially fatal. Morbid obesity is a condition in which the body is at least 100 pounds over its normal body mass resulting in a body mass index (BMI) greater than 40. Individuals with morbid obesity venture in many cases beyond the point at which they can engage in any activity at all. This makes it almost impossible for them to lose weight except through shear starvation. Eventually, they become burdensome to themselves and others because of their inability to access common utilities such as a toilet seat, wheel chair, airplane seat or even an automobile. Quite often with morbidly obese individuals, special consideration must be given to transport and contain them in an emergency. Because of their enormous fat accumulation, it becomes almost impossible to perform emergency cardiac life support or CPR on morbidly obese individuals.

6. Substance Abuse

Even though the rate of obesity is increasing worldwide and is especially high in the United States, the unpopular stigma of this condition continues to prevail. Indeed, being overweight is not in today's society a popular state. Those who are obese tend to be looked upon as second-class citizens. Some even believe overweight individuals to be of lower intelligence than normal individuals. Obese children tend to be bullied and harassed in school. Obese individuals are also considered by some as being a burden upon society especially in terms of health economics and social subsistence programs. As we shall see in the next section, obesity prevails among impoverished and poorly education persons, a factor which tends to place an untoward social marker on this condition.

There is no doubt, given the way that obese individuals are perceived that they can develop deep seated anxieties, apprehensions and chronic depression. In fact, depression and anxiety are very common among obese individuals. Although depression itself can be a serious condition leading often to notions of suicide, it can also evolve into more insidious behavior not the least of which may include substance abuse. In fact, depression is actually the leading cause of substance abuse. Alcohol and drugs are abused excessively by depressed individuals to help overcome their anxieties. These are narcotic substances that offer temporary feelings of euphoria, happiness and fullness of life. But withdrawal from alcohol and drugs can cause the underlying state of depression to become even more severe. Aside from this is that long-term abuse of these substances not only exacerbates the obese condition, but also results in other even more dangerous health risks.

C. Chapter Summary

Obesity is a condition that can lead to serious medical complications and even death. Insulin resistance resulting from obesity can cause a condition known as Type 2 Diabetes. Several types of carcinoma or neoplasms such as stomach cancer, pancreatic cancer and colon cancer are very common among those suffering from Type 2 Diabetes. Obesity can also lead to hypertension or high blood pressure which can cause strokes and heart attacks. Kidney disease can also be caused by obesity from an increase in blood sugar levels. High cholesterol levels resulting from obesity can cause the formation of gallstones leader to inflammation of the gallbladder. Over a long period of time, because of the extra weight carried by obese individuals, this can cause excessive wear and tear and eventual destruction of cartilage around the hip and knee joints through a condition known as osteoarthritis. Elevated heart and breathing resulting from the need for more blood oxygen among obese individuals also interfere with normal sleep.

The threat of obesity is equally as dangerous as obesity itself. Many individuals will combat their fear of being obese by acquiring certain psychotic behaviors meant to protect themselves from its onset. Some may starve themselves into a dangerous predisposition known as anorexia nervosa. Others still may go for long periods without food followed intermittently by binge eating. These individuals will periodically engorge themselves voraciously, consuming large quantities of food which they immediately purge through self-induced vomiting in a condition known as bulimia. Long-term fasting to avoid being fat can result in malnutrition from vitamin and mineral deficiency. It can also lead to a dangerous accumulation of ketones from the metabolism of stored fat through a condition known as ketosis.

The depression and psychosis associated with obesity can lead to behaviors that can make the problem even worse. Obese individuals in a denial state can adopt a sedentary life style which can lead to morbid obesity. Conditions that are a common state among obese individuals include anxiety and depression. These can lead to compensatory behaviors such as alcoholism and drug abuse.

Key Points:

1. Obesity is associated with insulin resistance leading to Type 2 Diabetes
2. Obesity is associated with certain types of cancer
3. Obesity is associated with high blood pressure leading to stroke and cardiovascular disease
4. Obesity is associated with gall stones and inflammation of the gallbladder
5. Obesity can lead to the destruction of the hip and knee joints
6. Obesity is associated with many sleep disorders including interrupted breathing or sleep apnea
7. Fear of being overweight or obese can lead to many defensive behaviors such a self-starvation or anorexia and binge eating such as bulimia which can lead to malnutrition and the accumulation of dangerous toxins
8. Obesity can lead to a sedentary life style
9. Obesity is associated with depression and anxiety which may result in the abuse of alcohol and drugs

Section II

Historical, Cultural and Economic Aspects of Obesity

Chapter 5--*Obesity through the Ages*

Obesity is not something that just recently happened to plague society. Because of the many advances in medical science and an increase in the cognitive awareness of obesity, its incidence and proliferation have begun to gain widespread attention, especially in recent years. But obesity has been around for a very long time. In fact, the ancient Egyptians first began regarding the condition as being unhealthy and actually developed programs to combat the condition, albeit, some of these, which included outright starvation and severe punishment, were considerably more problematic. The ancient Aztecs believed that obesity was a divine punishment or curse from the gods and would shun those who were afflicted by it accordingly. On the other hand, some Ancient African cultures believed that it was necessary to over feed or engorge a young mother in preparation for giving birth. Many ancient tribal cultures would combat famine by eating large amounts of food to store fat and thus became obese much like a bear would do before its winter hibernation.

Obesity first became acknowledged as a disease by the Greeks. In fact, the Greek physician Hippocrates, considered as being the father of medicine, discovered that there was a much higher incidence of sudden death, especially at a younger age, among individuals who were obese. Consequently, he began keeping extensive journals and logs of his findings. As a result of his research obesity became classified as a serious medical condition requiring immediate interventional management. Despite the findings and teachings of Hippocrates, however, superstition and misinformation about obesity continued through the middle ages during which treatment for the condition became often illogical and bazaar. Among the treatments was bloodletting, magic potions, steam therapy and ... just about everything but what would really successfully resolve the condition.

At some point during the middle ages, not only in Europe but also in East Asia, it was noted that most of the prominent leaders, politicians and wealthy individuals were obese. This later evolved into the notion that obesity was a sign of wealth, status and importance. Consequently, many people, even those who were impoverished became obese, perhaps to gain access to certain privileges or to gain favor with those of privilege. But obesity in the privileged class was more a function of gluttony, greed and excess than of any cultural or political notion. People of wealth and power during those times did very little for themselves, but instead had their work done by slaves, conscripts or servants from the impoverished population groups.

It is interesting to note that obesity appears to be more prevalent among the industrialized nations of the world than among those whose economies are based largely upon farming and agriculture. Industrialization developed much more rapidly in the European and Western civilizations where obesity is statistically higher. This is not a surprising development considering that industrialized nations are more readily able to provide for themselves. Obesity is also more prevalent in those nations whose governments are based on democracy and or rule of law than by those whose economies are suppressed by central ruling factions such as dictatorships and oligarchies. In fact, during the Middle Ages, famine and starvation was very high because of the absence of a central means of producing and distributing foods. Instead, most of the population, which was ruled locally by lords, barons and kings, was busy gathering provisions for their masters. This resulted in many local uprisings, a high crime rate and even outright war.

Even religion somehow plays a part in the prevalence of obesity; although it is not clear why accept that most religious philosophies tend to be highly disciplined against practices that often suppress the onset of obesity such as smoking and alcoholism. But, most of these notions are highly controversial.

A. War, Famine and Survival

When we think of war, it is a deplorable notion that also conjures fears of famine and death and thus increases our natural propensity for survival. During periods of war, massive resources are accumulated and used to support armies while at the same time these resources are wasted in the destructive path of war. War results almost invariably in nutritional rationing. It can also contribute to famine and all of the defensive behaviors that result such as hoarding foods, consuming foods high in carbohydrates and saturated fats and doing whatever is necessary to survive in the short-run.

1. War and Obesity

For as long as the human race has existed on earth, at one time or another, it was at war. There is significant archeological evidence to suggest that ancient tribes engaged frequently in fierce wars. These were very likely waged for the control of territories perceived as rich and abundant with sources of food. Indeed, most wars, even today, are fought to achieve some measure of control over natural resources—to survive. In many other cases, wars are the product unfortunately of greed, corruption and the lure of power. In ancient times, wars were fought primarily for food and fear of famine. Today, they are fought for resources such as oil and natural gas, again to be used in order the make the resources of survival more accessible.

They say that an army walks on its stomach or perhaps a navy then floats on its stomach. In either case one cannot fight a war without food. A warrior must be fed in order to survive the harsh and brutal character of war. But, unlike the diet that would be consumed by any normal individual, a soldier must eat very much like a modern athlete. Commanders in the battlefield have struggled throughout history with effective ways of nourishing their armies. The Romans were quite sophisticated at feeding their armies, providing entire legions of hunters and gatherers to keep their armies strong in battle. The Romans were among the first, in fact, to recognize the value of certain foods. They knew that foods rich in fat were essential to armies sent to fight in the cold, northern areas of Europe. They also recognized that foods high carbohydrates gave their armies sustained energy for long marches through rugged terrain.

The reader may wonder at this point just what war has to do with obesity. War actually results in at least two predispositions for obesity. First of all, a soldier may operate for years in harsh environments. A diet high in carbohydrates and fat would be sustained throughout this period. As long as the soldier remains active, these high concentrations could be effectively metabolized. Many soldiers return home, leave the military or retire, but do not necessarily alter their acquired dietary habits. If they become less active, but sustain the diet they were accustomed do in their military capacity, they can eventually become obese. Many studies, in fact, have shown a high rate of obesity among retired military personnel and even active military personnel who are reassigned from combat to support roles. Throughout history, in fact, high rates of obesity prevailed among soldiers after long periods in combat roles.

Yet another link between military activity and obesity is stress. Early in this book we discovered how stress can cause obesity by the release of the molecule *neuropeptide Y* which is known to cause an increase in the number of fat cells in the body. Stress is a fact of military life. Indeed, the prospect of going to battle in war is a source of severe anxiety, stress and even depression. This is the case even among the best-trained and most highly disciplined soldiers. The anticipation of injury or death in any situation can have long-term consequences upon the physiological makeup of the body.

It was not until after World War II that scientist began studying the link between war and the many post-war medical conditions suffered by veterans. For decades, the phrase post-traumatic stress disorder (PTSD) was used to describe the behavioral and clinical manifestations experienced by combat veterans. This resulted in an untoward stigma derived from ignorance and lack of information about the condition. As a result many affected veterans were shunned as cowards or as being weak. Described originally as a psychological condition, PTSD is now considered a serious clinical disease that can lead to many medical conditions including obesity. PTSD can also lead to alcoholism and drug abuse, both of which can contribute to obesity. In fact, studies have shown that the rate of obesity even among active duty military personnel always seems to increase during war time, but there appears to be no causal relationship except that the common thread that runs through every experience of war is stress.

2. Famine, Survival and Obesity

It is very difficult to understand perhaps how famine can have any relationship to obesity, but the link is very real and quite strong. For example, during World War II, there was so much destruction that literally millions of people died of shear starvation, especially in Europe and Russia. Many who survived developed altered states about their attitudes towards food. They considered it absolutely incomprehensible to waste anything. This led to an adoptive behavior in which everything cooked was eaten regardless of whether or not hunger was present. A life time of this obsessive-compulsive behavior led eventually to obesity.

Most individuals will alter their behavior in response to fear and the fear of famine, especially after having endured it before can conjure many types of obsessive behavior. Many who fear the onset of famine will hoard large amounts of food high in concentrated carbohydrates and fat. When they discover that the famine will not come after all they then proceed to consume this food so that it is not wasted.

Among ancient tribal cultures, hunters and gatherers would accumulate food high in fat content. Many scientists believe that this may have resulted in the evolution of a so called "Thrifty Gene" that is considered a heredity cause of obesity among descendents of these tribal cultures even today. Because there was no way to preserve the foods for long periods, ancient tribes would consume fatty foods in great quantities to prepare themselves for winter during which food would be scarce. Most would become obese but only temporarily for the purpose of survival. During winter time, provided that activity levels were significantly reduced, the enormous fat stores in the body was gradually metabolized quite the way bears and other hibernating creatures would use stored energy. It was later discovered that salt could extend the life of certain meats, so long-term storage became possible. But, this resulted in an over-accumulation of salt in the body, hypertension and obesity.

B. The Industrial and Technological Revolutions

For thousands of years, up to and including the Middle Ages, very little had been accomplished to improve life. But much of this was the consequence of war. In fact, war became even more prevalent after the fall of the Roman Empire. Tribal cultures prevailed and society became largely disjointed and scattered. This led to an abrupt decline in the development of technology leading to the so called "Dark Ages" or Medieval Times. The Dark Ages lasted for about 1000 years from 500 A.D to 1500 A.D. Although the military complex certainly became gradually more sophisticated during this period, primarily through the advent of iron, everything else was held constant. Obesity still prevailed, but primarily among the wealthy. Everyone else remained thin from hard work and very little, if anything, to eat. By the very nature of society, physical activity was plentiful and food was scarce, but only by necessity. Because food had to be either hunted or grown, it was neither readily available nor even easy to acquire. It was also difficult to preserve food, so hunting was a frequent, highly active undertaking. Even those who didn't or couldn't hunt were busy tending to the fields gathering crops or preparing meals.

It suddenly dawned upon wise members of society that war was not the answer to survival. It was reasoned instead that trade and barter were much more logical and productive undertakings. Indeed, what one nation or tribe had could be traded for what another had and intertribal or intercommunity equilibrium would prevail. So, instead of destroying each other's resources societies began to share them. Profitability and abundance eventually began to permeate society and peace prevailed at least long enough for everyone to begin thinking about things other than survival. They were still active and busy, but mostly at building, inventing and developing. In fact, trade yielded not only to an abundance of shared resources but also knowledge. This led beginning in about the 15th century, to the Renaissance. The term "Renaissance" is actually French for rebirth and refers to a revival of thought and innovation.

The Renaissance movement gave birth to a litany of ideas, cultural improvements and radical innovations during a period that spanned almost three hundred years. Although art and architecture were predominantly affected, the massive development in the ship-building industry during this period led to an acceleration of world trade and economic growth. Soon the integration of ideas among trading cultures led in about 1800 A.D. to the great Industrial Revolution. It was during this period that life gave in to invention and hard work to technology. It was now possible to produce and deliver goods and services much faster and further. Instead of hunting and gathering food, this would eventually become available through central stores and establishments. As a consequence of these developments, of course, more leisure time became available.

Having to contend less with survival and more with leisure and self-fulfillment, society began searching for more creative ways to remain active. With very little else to do after work but play, many engaged in organized sports. Despite this, however, technology continued to advance, almost geometrically through the 1800's and 1900's. Up until the late 1800's, the major modes of transportation included the horse and anything driven by a horse, the bicycle and, of course, walking and running. Horses were a common mode of transportation but were expensive and high-maintenance. In about 1885, the first bicycle was introduced and, although an excellent source of physical activity, was not nearly as effective as a horse through rugged, unpaved terrain.

The beginning of the end of serious physical activity may well have been inaugurated in 1891 when the first automobile or horseless carriage was introduced by the French. The Pennard-Levassor as the first car was known completely changed the landscape of human endeavor. Soon, hundreds of thousands of automobiles were made available to the public. At the same time, Thomas Edison was busy making life even more convenient with his investon of, among other things, the light bulb. The car, the light bulb and, of course, other practical uses of electricity ushered in the Technological Revolution. Up until about 1950, technology had not yet overcome the pursuit of leisurely physical activity. Then there came radio followed by the television.

With cars available to keep us off our feet and radio and television to keep us at home, what else could possibly hinder our means of staying active? Well, probably the greatest invention of modern times was the personal computer. With the introduction of the personal computer in about 1980, if the owners of these devices were not watching television, they would simply work on their computers. In fact, the personal computer eventually became a source of entertainment so instead of sitting to watch television one would sit and play computer games. As a result of all of these extraordinary technological developments, an insidious proliferation of the passive-sedentary life style prevailed and the rate of obesity began to rise geometrically, especially in the industrialized world.

There is extraordinary correlating evidence to suggest that world industrialization has led to an increase in obesity. In fact, there is a direct correlation between the wealth of nations, those having large industrial complexes, and their rate of obesity. In the industrialized nations, not only has leisure time been largely replaced with access to modern technology such as personal computers, but hunting, gathering and cooking has been largely replaced by the abundance, variety and centralized availability of food. Thanks to the speed and efficiency of international trade, where food was once derived from local sources, it could now be obtained all over the world. This resulted in drastic changes in the dietary habits of society.

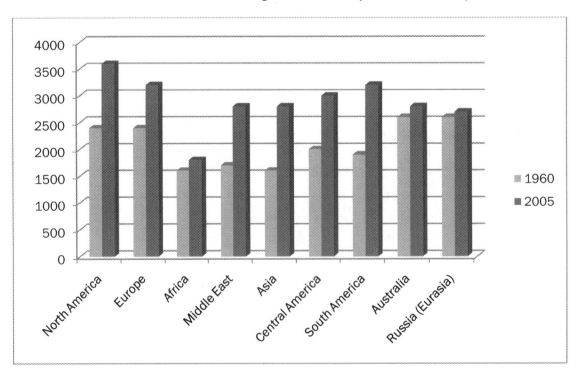

Figure 4: Average Daily Consumption in Kilocalories

It soon became possible for Americans to consume foods from Japan, Russia, China, India, etc.; and, in the converse, the latter countries could do likewise with American foods. The diverse variety of foods that became available led to dietary experimentation and the proliferation of hundreds of different types of restaurants, especially in the culturally diverse populations of the United States.

It is believed that obesity may be linked to the evolution of technology as indicated by an increase in the average amount of calories (kilocalories) consumed. In most continents between 1960 and 2005 there was a significant increase in caloric intake per capita, due largely to an increase in world trade initiatives and resulting industrialization. Except for the continents of Africa, Australia and Eurasia (primarily Russia), obesity has risen significantly since 1960 as reflected in **Figure 4** above.

With resources readily available and leisure time relegated to watching television and playing computer games, a rapid change in lifestyle began to permeate the more affluent nations. The highest rate of obesity as of the publication of this book is in the United States, but this doesn't necessarily mean that we are a gluttonous nation. Again, rates of obesity are determined by a combination of factors including the availability, accessibility and variety of foods. It is also determined by factors that may not be within our total control. For example, during the late 1800's and on through the early 1900's, the industrialization of America led to a massive migration of those in rural areas to the urban complex where jobs were most prevalent. The great cities provided very little, if any, outlets for an active lifestyle. Moreover, the higher crime rates, as well as industrial pollutants and noise levels in urban areas kept most individuals home after work. Instead of walking or riding a bicycle to work, it was much safer to take taxi or mass transit conveyances. As a consequence of this virtually uncontrollable lifestyle, obesity prevailed.

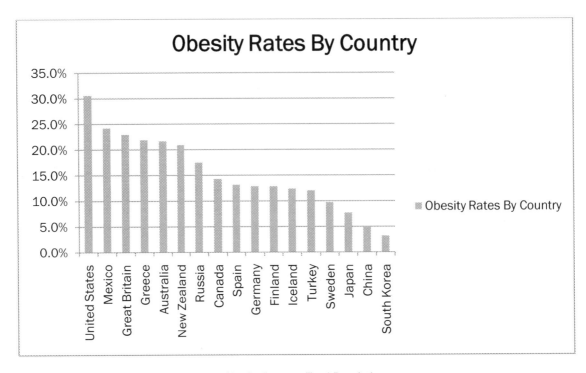

Figure 5: Average Obesity Rates to Total Population

Even though food became readily accessible and available among industrialized nations, it had to be massed produced and shipped to all parts of the world. Instead of hobby and family farms, massive crop farms and ranches would become the major source of food. These massive complexes required radical changes in the way food was handled and processed. In order to avoid the loss of large fields of crops farmers would use toxic pesticides. Meats and other processed foods would be injected with steroids, additives and preservatives. One example, which has had a significant impact upon obesity, especially in the United States, is a process known as hydrogenation. With this process, unsaturated fatty acids such as those contained in vegetable oils are altered atomically by bonding their carbon atoms with hydrogen atoms. This process makes the unsaturated fats behave like saturated fats, thus allowing them to harden like butter or lard when cooled. Hydrogenation was discovered 1897 by French chemist Paul Sabatier and is used to increase the shelf life of unsaturated oils and any products containing these oils. It also helps to preserve their flavor. But, just like the saturated fats, because hydrogenated, unsaturated fats make the latter become essentially like their saturated counterpart, their consumption can lead to obesity. Hydrogenation also yields a byproduct known as trans-fatty acids or the so called "twisted molecule". Trans-fatty acids act like toxins that tend to counteract rather than to improve the health benefits of certain foods.

C. Time is the New Enemy

Among the most significant influences upon the rate of obesity, especially among modern industrialized nations is time. Prior to the Industrial Revolution, most families stayed within close proximity of their homes and carefully divided daily chores among its members. Some family members would hunt while others would tend to livestock, till and sew crops. Still others would prepare and cook meals as well as to clean and maintain the dwelling. As the industrial revolution evolved, family members would migrate away from rural areas to the industrial urban areas where jobs were readily available. At first, only one family member would work abroad while the others would stay home and keep house. But, as the cost of living began to increase and the work force demanded more financial success and growth, soon all adult family members would seek work where it was available, in many cases, just to survive. Today both spouses usually work while their children are held at day care centers or with a baby sitter. When they would come home for work, there would scarcely be enough time to cook and bond before bed time and another day at work. The only time available for any active lifestyle was during the weekends when most family members would rest after a long and arduous work week.

The constraint of time works against us in at least two ways. First is that it takes time to be physically active. Physicians, in fact, recommend at least one hour per day of vigorous exercise such as jogging, bicycling or walking. Although younger people are more likely to jog or ride a bike, as they get older this is relegated to walking and one must walk at least three miles to obtain the same benefits as jogging one mile. Thus, instead of one hour, one must exercise perhaps as much as three hours per day in order to avoid becoming obese. The second imposition is that a lack of sufficient time gives little or no opportunity to prepare organized meals. Consequently, more people than ever before are eating out often as much as three days out of each weak at three take-out meals per day.

D. Ignorance is Bliss

Prior to the proliferation of international trade, food was gathered largely from local, primarily autonomous sources. There were few if any central food distribution systems and local grocers were stocked usually with food from nearby farms and ranches. More importantly, is that people ate what they did without really understanding the nutritional value of foods. Consequently, many people became obese from eating foods rich in carbohydrates and saturated fats. Matters did not improve much after the Industrial Revolution. In fact, the Industrial Revolution ushered in the mass production and distribution of foods, not only from local sources, but also from countries around the world through international trade. Foods were now being produced on a much larger scale and then distributed to local grocers from great distances. As a result of these mass production innovations, new concerns began to emerge, especially in regard to how foods are prepared, preserved and stored before distribution.

The Industrial Revolution made food so abundant and readily available, especially among developed nations, that thousands of restaurants began to sprout and more and more people began to explore the variety of cuisines that were now available. But, this became much to the exclusion of any thought about their nutritional value or even whether or not the foods were safe to eat. Many of the foods were rich in spices and preservatives quite to the point that they became health risks. Up until the late 1800's very little if anything was known about the dangers of saturated fats. Many foods were prepared using lard and butter. Without any information to the contrary, people ate heartily on these highly unhealthy, nutritionally weak foods.

As with so many developments over time profitability too often overshadowed practicality and safety. Consequently, new laws emerged to protect and inform consumers about the health risks of food beginning as early as 1906 with the Food and Drug Act. The Food and Drug Act of 1906 was also known as the "Wiley" act after Harvey Washington Wiley, whose intense campaign against the questionable practices of food manufacturers and distributors led to sweeping changes in the way foods were prepared and delivered to the public. Many more laws were enacted thereafter resulting eventually in strict guidelines on the way foods were classified, labeled and even dated for consumption. After 1938 all foods required expiration dates. Then in 1966, the Fair Packaging and Labeling Act required that all packaged food be labeled with net contents, product identity as well as the names of the manufacturer, packer and distributor. Although restaurants were excluded from the act, the Nutrition labeling and Education Act of 1990 required most foods to be labeled with a schedule of its contents, including calories, percentage of daily nutritional requirements, etc.

Despite the many laws and regulations enacted to inform the lay public about the nutritional content and value foods, ignorance of these factors still prevails today. Most do not fully understand nor even take the time to evaluate food labels. Imagine, for example, preparing a four-course meal for guests and, in so doing, calculating precisely the percentage of USDA (United Stated Department of Agriculture) daily allowance, also known as RDA (Recommended Daily Allowance) for certain essential vitamins, carbohydrates, protein and fat. It is usually only when confronted with obesity that the nutritional value and caloric content of foods really begin to matter.

E. Obesity Can be Contagious

When we think of a contagious disease, we are usually referring to something brought about by communicable viruses and bacteria. But, social interaction and behavior can also be contagious in ways that may surprise the reader. Indeed, the rapid rise and proliferation of obesity, especially during the past 100 years following the Industrial Revolution could not simply have evolved from self-imposed eating habits and growing lack of activity. Studies have shown in fact, that not only did obesity prevail more in the urban than rural areas, but the rate at which obesity had increased was much higher with urban than with rural population groups. This led to the supposition that obesity was somehow contagious—that if one individual was obese then it is likely that close friends, co-workers and relatives would also become obese.

The seemingly absurd notion that obesity is contagious was actually proven based upon a study of more than 12,000 people from 1971 to 2003. This study, the results of which were published in the New England Journal of Medicine, revealed that persons were most likely to become obese when a friend, associate or relative was obese. In fact, the mere association with an obese person increased one's likelihood of becoming obese by about 57%. This led to a new catch phrase that certain behaviors can be "Socially Contagious". It is well known how certain behaviors can be socially transmitted. A good example is how fads and trends are introduced and permeate into society. Advertising has evolved into a very successful source of socially contagious behavior. This trend grew rapidly with the advent of television and now the internet or worldwide web.

F. The Influence of Art, Cinema and Television

The notion that behavior is contagious follows also from the influence of television and motion picture celebrities. Indeed, many of us tend to mimic or assimilate the behaviors of our favorite movie and television stars many of whom are (or were) obese. These include such popular actors as Charles Laughton, Chill Wills, Raymond Burr, Jackie Gleason, Theodore Bikel, Peter Ustinov, Curt Jergens, Eli Wallach, Slim Pickens, Telly Savalas, Marlon Brando, John Belushi, John Candy, Kirstie Alley, Elvis Presley, John Goodman, Queen Latifah, Orson

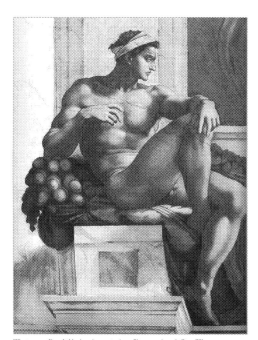

Wells, Jack Black, W. C. Fields and others. Obesity also prevailed among the highly influential U.S. presidents such as John Adams, Grover Cleveland, William Howard Taft, Teddy Roosevelt and Lyndon Johnson, among world leaders such as Winston Churchill, Mao Tse Tung, Nikita Krushchev and great musicians such as Luciano Pavorotti, Burl Ives and Louis Armstrong.

Even before television, radio and the cinema, the cultural influence of obesity transcended the community in many other forms such as sculpture, paintings and the theater. In art, human figures, especially those of woman, were portrayed as robust and, by modern standards, probably overweight. But this was not necessarily a reflection of reality. Instead, artists painted or sculpted human figures to emphasize certain

Figure 6: Michelangelo, "Ignudo 18: The Ignudi", Cistine Chapel

anatomical features. This was especially evident in many of the renaissance paintings of Michelangelo, Raphael, Peter Paul Rubens and Leonardo da Vinci. These artists painted men with vastly exaggerated muscular-skeletal features to emphasize strength. The head of the male was small in relation to the size of his body to show that strength and vigor were more important than the power of the brain (Figure 6). Female anatomy was especially exaggerated in art, but not necessarily to show that women were overweight or obese or to poke fun at obesity. Nude paintings of woman generally emphasized the abdomen and buttocks, as in Ruben's "Venus at a Mirror" (Figure 7), in tribute to female reproduction and fertility. Female breasts were often portrayed as excessively large in proportion to the body and the female abdomen or "Venus Mound" distended and rounded to further emphasize this celebration of female sexuality.

The exaggeration of human anatomy by artists, although quite deliberately intended euphemistically to emphasize certain human attributes, may have in many ways actually influenced human behavior. Just as modern advertising tends to alter our perceptions of reality, so too did art because it was among the only visual references to popular culture prior to the advent of photography and electronic media. Painting and sculpture were like modern billboard conveyances, offering society a virtual window to other realities. In the absence of any other reference to the contrary, other than local, autonomous cultures, paintings and sculptures depicted how people may have appeared in other cultures. Consequently, if a female appeared busty with large buttocks in art, perhaps many who viewed the art may have themselves assimilated the anatomical attributes that art conveyed. In this case, obesity may have evolved as a function of social convention and behavior rather than self-indulgence.

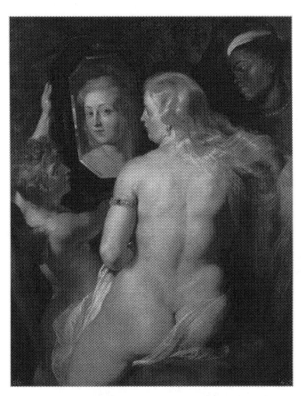

Figure 7: Rubens "Venus at a Mirror"

G. Religious and Philosophical Implications of Obesity

Among the lessons of philosophy and religion is that anything done in moderation is acceptable as long as it does not harm oneself or one's neighbor. But, anything done in excess whether harmful or not is considered sinful or unacceptable. These philosophical guidelines presuppose, however, that harmful or excessive behaviors are within one's immediate and unequivocal control. Many believe that obesity is a product of excessive-compulsive behavior, gluttony and/or greed; but, this is certainly not the case among most who suffer from obesity. A more accurate predisposition to obesity may simply be neglect, aberrant metabolism or physiological handicap. Neglect can be modified by correction, but physiology and metabolism are almost entirely out of one's control. So how does philosophy or, for that matter, even religion deal with the notion that one's condition is the consequence of a physiological or metabolic handicap?

There are many who believe that religion and philosophy are not the products of divine will, but rather the embodiment of an elaborate system of cognitive values intended to regulate the behavior of individuals. Proponents of this notion argue that, in the absence of philosophy and/or religion, anarchy would prevail and society could never develop into a civilization. Whether or not this is true, obesity has prevailed despite any real or perceived philosophical or religious convention. In fact, some believe that philosophy and religion may have actually fostered the development of obesity. This follows from the notion that food is the essence of life itself.

It is clear that food is the substance of life and its existence in nature whether naturally derived or endowed upon us by a higher spiritual power, is considered a gift consistent with that of life itself. In the Judeo-Christian faith, food is often held up as a symbol of spiritual strength. The Christian faith holds food as sacred and the lack thereof as the abandonment of God. This was underscored when the power of God was manifest in one of the legendary miracles of Jesus Christ. With only a loaf of bread and two fish, Jesus conjured enough food to feed some 5,000 followers. But, many subscribe this to the adage, "If you teach a [man] to fish, [he] would be fed for life." Nevertheless, it states in the Christian bibles, "Man shall not live by bread alone, but by everything that proceeds out of the mouth of the Lord" (Deuteronomy 8.3, Christian transliteration of the original Aramaic and Greek texts). But these examples have also been interpreted to refer, not to food, but how eating food is likened to hearing, obeying and disseminating the teachings of God.

On the other hand, the Christian bibles also state in Proverbs 23:20-22, "Be not among drunkards or among gluttonous eaters of meat, for the drunkard and the glutton will come to poverty, and slumber will clothe them with rags." This verse is used frequently by vegetarians to support their dietary philosophy, but it does not necessarily mean the exclusion of alcohol and meat. For example, it says, in 1 Timothy 4:1-4, "… some shall depart from faith … commanding to abstain from meats which God hath created to be received with thanksgiving of them which believe and know the truth." Moreover, we also know that fish is a type of meat and Jesus fed thousands with it; and, in 1 Timothy 5:23, it states, "Drink no longer water, but a little wine for thy stomach's sake and thine often infirmities". There are many more verses which are used often either to justify or to condemn obesity. Even exercise is not immune from biblical reference. In 1 Timothy 8:8, for example, it reads "For bodily exercise profiteth little …"

Some religions like Buddhism, at least in certain derivatives of this faith, foster the belief that obesity is a symbol of health, wealth and abundance of life. They portray the icon of their beliefs with a sort of "pot-bellied Buddha". But Buddhism is really not a deity-based religion. In fact, Buddhists do not generally believe in an invisible, omnipotent being as do the Christians, Jews and Muslims. Buddhism is almost exclusively a philosophy-based religion which advocates self-control and discipline, moderation and respect. In many ways, Buddhism is like the Hindu faith in which life is determined, not by the will of an invisible being, but by the inner being or by the self. With this in mind, any patterns of obesity among Buddhist and Hindu believers are more a function of culture than of spiritual belief.

Religion and philosophy are not necessarily sources of obesity per se, but may in some way influence the onset of obesity by the impressions they may impose upon human behavior. Indeed, if the way an individual appears or behaves is philosophically or spiritually endowed, then it must be so; but, this all depends largely upon how these dictums are interpreted or, more importantly, how they are conveyed by influential clerics and philosophical leaders. While obesity may result from certain philosophical or religious influences, there are other influences that may have the opposite effect. Fasting is a common practice among several philosophical and religious cultures. Fasting, in this case, is intended to give the body a chance to purge any toxins or "evil spirits", as it were, and to renew the body's vigor and energy. Although fasting can result in rapid, often dangerous weight loss, it can also result in an increase in body mass over time. The reader may recall in the previous chapter how the body's starvation stimuli can substantially lower thermic and basal metabolism. At this reduced state, when the fasting period is over, the return to a normal diet can result in an increase in body mass because fewer calories will be burned.

H. Chapter Summary

Obesity is not something that just crept into society in recent years. On the contrary, society has in some way struggled with this problem for thousands of years, perhaps even during the age of ancient tribal cultures. Nevertheless, only recently has society actually come to grips with its many underlying causes. Through the ages, war and famine have played a significant role in the proliferation of obesity. War is wrought with stress and anxiety, both of which contribute to obesity; and, famine conjures many obsessive behaviors that can lead to obesity. The advancement of civilization through international trade, innovation and technology has contributed significantly to the proliferation of obesity. This has evolved, especially among, wealthy, industrialized nations, from a technologically induced reduction in activity, the ease of accessibility, variety and availability of food, urban migration, reduction in leisure time and the influence of the media, arts, religion and philosophy.

Key Points:

1. Stress resulting from the horrors of war can lead to obesity
2. The physical and psychological effects of famine can lead to obesity
3. The Industrial and Technological Revolutions resulted in decreased activity and increased consumption, based upon variety, quantity and availability of food
4. Industrial food processing techniques such as hydrogenation may impose health risks including obesity
5. Obesity may be considered "Socially Contagious" in that one individual may become obese if he/she is closely related to someone who is obese
6. Obesity may be significantly influenced by the arts
7. Obesity is linked to many religious and philosophical principles and practices
8. Fasting may result in obesity when normal diets are resumed at the lower metabolic rate

Chapter 6—*the Demographics of Obesity*

We have seen how obesity can be influenced by philosophy, religion, social relationships and even the media; but, the rate of obesity itself varies significantly across cultural, national and ethnic origins. Although one might expect the impoverished, so called "Third-World" cultures to have a lower incidence of obesity, quite the contrary, the incidence is similar and, in some cases even higher, than in the wealthier cultures, although limited to certain ethnic, cultural and national origins. Whereas the incidence of obesity in wealthy cultures may be a function of readily accessible nutrition, the nutrients consumed by those in certain impoverished cultures are likely much higher in fat and carbohydrates for energy metabolism and storage. But, overall, obesity has the highest incidence as well as the highest rate of increase over time among wealthy and industrialized regions of the world.

Obesity has actually become rather a pandemic, spreading worldwide with more than one billion persons being overweight and about a third of these considered obese or morbidly obese. We have noted in the previous chapter that, although obesity has prevailed to some extent throughout the ages, it became a serious, almost explosive problem following the Industrial and Technological revolutions. The two principal predispositions to obesity introduced by these important historical events are an increased variety and availability of foods. Consequently, and not surprisingly, obesity is highest among geographic regions having the highest concentration of wealth, those which are heavily industrialized and those having the capability of engaging in international trade. It is also no surprise that the nations regarded as being the wealthiest and most powerful in the world such as the United States, Great Britain and Canada have the highest obesity rates.

Just as obesity appears to be higher among industrialized geographic regions than among agricultural or non-industrial regions, it is also higher per capita (per person) among urban than among rural population centers. This follows logically from the fact that food is considerably more accessible in the urban centers. Because of the high concentration of populations in urban areas, there is certainly a more efficient and, of course, a greater abundance of food centers and distribution mechanisms than one would find in rural areas. So, does this lead us to the conclusion that the principal cause of obesity is the availability of food? Not necessarily. The abundance and variety of foods is clearly a factor in the proliferation of obesity worldwide; but, it is very important for the reader to understand that wealth and industry go hand in hand with virtually all of the many predispositions to obesity discussed in **Chapter 3** of this text. Indeed, the industrialized, wealthy nations have a much higher incidence of the many causes of obesity. Because jobs are more readily available in these regions, stress levels are higher, time available for leisurely activity is much lower, substance abuse related to stress and anxiety is much higher, poor eating habits related to job-induced time constraints are much higher and the list goes on.

A. Obesity, Race and Ethnicity

It is very difficult to construct a logical argument which suggests that obesity is a functional result of one's race, ethnicity or origin. The fact that an individual is either White or Black, Asian or Hispanic really does not seem to relate to any physical predispositions or standards of human development. So then why are there such wide deviations in the rate of obesity among ethnic and racial classifications? To answer this question, we must examine each classification carefully in terms of the many other factors that cause obesity which we learned in the **Section I** of this text.

1. Standards of Population Classification

There is often a great deal of confusion and controversy when attempting to classify various population groups. Some like to use race as a baseline classification while others like the term ethnicity. But race and ethnicity are really two very distinct terms. Race refers to a much broader classification of population groups and distinguishes such groups by biological and physical similarities. In general, there are actually only six classifications of race while ethnicity, which is more akin to culture than to physical characteristics, consist of only two different classifications. These are summarized in **Table XI** below.

Table XI: Differentiation of Race and Ethnicity Standards		
Classification	Standard	Definition
American Indian or Alaskan Native	Race	Anyone having descended from the original peoples of North, Central and South America
Asian (Mongoloid or Mongolic)	Race	Those who are descendants of the original peoples of East and Southeast Asia, as well as the Indian subcontinent, including Cambodia, Vietnam, India, Japan, Korea, Malaysia, Pakistan, the Philippines or Indonesia and Thailand
Black or African-American (Congroid and Capoid)	Race	Anyone having origins in any of the black racial groups of Africa
Native Hawaiian or Pacific Islander	Race	Those who are descendants of the original peoples of Hawaii,

Table XI: Differentiation of Race and Ethnicity Standards		
Classification	Standard	Definition
		Guam, Samoa or other Pacific Island
White (Caucasian or Caucasoid, Anglo-Saxon)	Race	Those who are descendants of the original peoples of Europe, the Middle East and North Africa
Australoid	Race	Includes those of Aboriginal descent in Australia and New Zealand
Hispanic or Latino	Ethnicity	Any person of Cuba, Mexico, South or Central America or other Spanish or cultural origin regardless of race
Non-Hispanic	Ethnicity	All other race classifications

Regardless of how populations are classified, the use of terms and standards to differentiate cultures, human physical characteristics and the like has become controversial at best; hence, this book makes no claims or distinctions about race and ethnicity nor offers any demarcations thereof. The intent by using such classifications to describe the incidence and prevalence of obesity is the show how the latter is in some way influenced by race and ethnicity. It is important to understand how and why obesity prevails more in one classification than in another. This can establish, in many respects scientifically, the etiological or physiological mechanism of obesity. We know, for example, that obesity is higher among Blacks than among Asians. What we do not know is why and can only speculate that it may have something to do with physical characteristics and diet.

2. Race and Poverty

For various reasons that are not clearly understood even today, obesity appears to prevail more in certain races and/or ethnic groups than others. For example, Blacks or African-Americans have the highest prevalence of obesity, especially among Black or African-American females. Many believe that this is a function of culture and economics. Only until recently have Blacks been racially confounded by discrimination. It is believed that this has contributed significantly to the economic suppression of African-Americans leading to a high rate of poverty within this classification. This rate of economic suppression has lead over many years to the migration of African-Americans into urbanized communities where jobs are more readily available. In general, there are more African-Americans living in urban areas than in rural areas of the United States. As already suggested, rates of obesity are much higher in urban than in rural areas for various reasons other than racial origin.

While there may be wide deviations in obesity rates across racial lines, this may have considerably less to do with race or ethnic origin than it does with how these origins have been influenced by culture and economics. For example, obesity appears to be higher among low income than among high income population groups. It is also higher among poorly educated that among well-educated individuals regardless of race. Many scientists believe that these factors tend to bear significant influences upon diet and activity. Impoverished and poorly educated individuals tend to be less active and consume foods higher in saturated fats and carbohydrates. Poorly educated individuals tend to be ignorant of the dietary significance of certain foods. Impoverished individuals will tend to purchase foods that are less expensive, yet more filling. Potatoes and pasta products and meats having high concentrations of saturated fats are far less expensive than foods rich in protein and unsaturated fats.

The reader may have noticed among race classifications that Hispanics or Latinos are not included; however, they are considered an ethnic classification. In fact, Hispanics, or those of Latin or Spanish origin, are actually considered White despite their skin color. Nevertheless, when it relates to statistical studies Hispanics are often distinguished from Whites in order to differentiate the study objective between cultural and socio-economic patterns of behavior. Having said this now, it is interesting to note that Hispanics have the second highest rate of obesity after Blacks. Coincidentally, this population group also has the second highest poverty rate. In fact, when we look comparatively at rates of poverty and corresponding rates of obesity in the U.S., the correlation is remarkably high as demonstrated in **Table XII** below.

Table XII: Correlation of Poverty and Obesity		
Race/Ethnicity	**Rate of Poverty**	**Rate of Obesity**
White	8.55%	17.01%
Asian-America	11.80%	19.16%
African-American	24.71%	27.33%
Hispanic	23.23%	27.01%

Source: NHANES 1999-2000; Centers for Disease Control Data 2006-2008

Among the principal reasons that obesity rates are high among the impoverished is based upon a theory known as *food insecurity*. This theory tends to help dispel the unusual paradox that prevails with the phenomenon of obesity among the poor. Food insecurity is a defensive behavior among the poor to obtain the most, not nutritional value, but hunger relief value, for the least cost. Unfortunately, many low cost foods such as pasta, potatoes and processed meats such as Spam, Prem and frankfurters or hot dogs are high in carbohydrates and saturated fats

3. Race and Political Suppression

From a global perspective it is also interesting to note that the rate of obesity among Blacks is less than among African-Americans. Again, this is largely a function of differences between the industrialized and non-industrialized, so called "Third-World" cultures. Then too, Asian-Americans tend to have a higher rate of obesity than Asians worldwide. In fact, Asians in general appear to have the lowest rate of obesity; however, the trend in obesity among Asians in recent years is actually highest among all the race classifications. This leads us to another interesting hypothesis, that obesity prevails less among politically suppressed and oppressed cultures than among free cultures. For example, only recently has China changed its political and economic landscape which for centuries had been ruled by communist suppression and restricted behaviors. Nations suppressed by centralized rule such as China and North Korea tend to focus the predominance of their gross domestic product upon military rather than upon socio-economic development. Consequently, those who live in these depressed environments tend to be rationed nutritionally because food availability and distribution is so highly regulated.

Over the past several years since the year 2000, major changes in the political landscape of China led to significant increases in the influence of Western culture, especially from corporate business interests in America, much of Europe and Great Britain. Consequently, the proliferation of industrial and economic culture, as well as significant increases in urbanization, has led to a rapid increase in the rate of obesity in this heavily populated nation. Where once, the thought of consuming American or for that matter, "Western" food was forbidden, there now prevail literally thousands of fast food restaurants dominated primarily by McDonald's and Kentucky Fried Chicken. This led to an abrupt change in the dietary and nutritional habits of a population whose primary source of food consisted of rice, poultry and fish. In terms of nutritional sophistication, in fact, the Chinese are now where the Western world had been around the turn of the 20th century, not because they are unsophisticated to be sure, but primarily because they were politically suppressed as a nation. The Chinese are fast beginning to realize that urbanization, industrialization, international trade and the resulting availability and variety of foods are fast beginning to introduce obesity as a major health issue in this culture.

Quite like China, the socio-economic changes that have occurred in Russia since the end of its reign as the Union of Soviet Socialist Republic (USSR) or the so called "Soviet Union" in 1991 led more and more to the proliferation of Western culture. Although there has been much controversy over its ethnic and racial classification, because Russia is considered part of the Asian continent, its people are considered largely Asian. On the other hand, many believe Russians to be White because of their physical characteristics in general. In either case, even

Russians are beginning to step into the obesity conundrum, not because of their race or ethnic classification, but because of their recent socio-economic development. So, whether we classify Russians as being White or Asian really doesn't matter except how they are being counted in either classification will influence statistical comparability.

B. Obesity and Cultural Origin

The notion that obesity may be a function of the political profile of certain cultures conjures the notion that governments can influence social behavior. In free political nations such as Canada, the United States, Japan, Great Britain and many other European nations, the rate of obesity is the highest in the world. But is this really because people are free to eat as much as they want and what they want? Indeed, are we suggesting here that the availability and variety of food are the real culprits in this growing global epidemic? If so, then are we asserting that humans have little or no self-control? On the contrary, behavior is not necessarily an autonomous condition. Behavior is either inherited, culturally (or politically) influenced or both. Indeed, we tend to behave as our ancestors did. Otherwise, we tend to behave in accordance with how we are influenced by the behavior of society in general. This was demonstrated by studies which show that obesity can actually be contagious.

1. The Three Worlds

In most Third-World cultures of the world, food is not nearly as readily available as in the wealthy, developed nations of the world. Indeed, in the United States, virtually every town having a population greater than 5,000 will likely have a large supermarket, several fast-food restaurants and many more quick-stop or overnight grocery markets. But, Third-World cultures are very much like the United States was during its pre-colonial development and migration. In this state, food was obtained through rigorous hunting and gathering activities which flourished only during warm seasons. Food preservation and storage did not exist and the death rate from famine and starvation was significantly high.

In order to understand the impact of culture upon obesity it is necessary to differentiate among the three levels of world culture. Most industrialized and developed nations of the world such as the United States, Japan and Great Britain, etc., are considered *First-World* cultures. First-World cultures are those that are highly urbanized and industrialized and those in which there is little if any proliferation of life-threatening, communicable diseases. *Second-World* cultures are those in which there is moderate industrial development and very few, if any, large urban centers. Second-World cultures are largely agricultural and rely heavily upon trade from the First-World cultures. Mexico, Nigeria and Thailand are examples of Second-World cultures. *Third-World* cultures, consisting of more than 70% of the world's population, are those in which there is little or no industrial development and the per capita income is less than $20 U.S. dollars per year. Most of Africa, some of the Middle East, Mongolia and much of Southeast Asia are considered Third-World.

It is very important for the reader to understand why cultures are so widely differentiated. The most obvious reason is geography. In many geographies of the world there are few, if any, indigenous natural resources by which a culture can engage in international trade. A large portion of Africa, for example, consists of desert and dense jungles. The Middle East is encompassed almost entirely of desert geology; however, the development of Middle Eastern nations has been fostered largely by its abundance of oil. Mongolia is primarily desert land and Southeast Asia, dense jungle. It is very difficult if not impossible to develop agricultural resources in either desert or jungle environments; however, the latter is rich in many resources used to develop pharmaceutical products. Because resources are scarce and international trade almost non-existent in Third-World cultures, they are governed generally by despotic, often violent rule marred by intermittent periods of revolution, war and genocide.

Even though the Third-World cultures are largely poor this has not precluded the onset of obesity. We've seen how poverty and lack of education can contribute to obesity in the First-World cultures. In similar fashion, lack of food and the behavioral consequences of food insecurity has also contributed to obesity in the Third-World cultures, but not to as great an extent since many in these cultures die of starvation, disease or from the consequences of war.

2. Food Culture

The prevalence of obesity is dependent as much upon the pattern of diet particular to a given culture as it is upon the availability and variety of food. There are many countries whose diets consist primarily of complex carbohydrates and fats, while still others whose diets are largely composed of proteins. In most Asian nations, rice, poultry and fish are the primary food staples. These are high protein diets whose regular consumption would generally not contribute to obesity. On the other hand, countries where foods such as beef, pork, potatoes, as well as high concentrations of milk and cheese are consumed will likely have the highest rates of obesity.

Despite the types of food that are consumed from country to country, probably the most significance influence upon food culture worldwide has been the advent and proliferation of the "Fast-Food" culture. This is especially true among the developed nations of the world where urbanization and modernization may actually have necessitated the need to rapidly access sources of food. The fast-food culture was actually derived from the rapid change in the cost of living requirements of families in the industrialized, First-World cultures. Instead of one bread-winner, the survival or sustained life-style of most families after the 1960's required that both spouses work. This left little or no time, or perhaps, no desire to prepare foods. Employers helped contribute to the problem by limiting their rest periods, often to just one hour per day divided into two 15-minute and one 30-minute rest period. Indeed, with these restrictions, it was convenient to grab a five-minute lunch at a local fast-food establishment.

The problem with the fast-food culture is not necessarily associated with convenience and availability. Instead, it is the content of the foods that poses the greatest influence upon obesity. Double burgers with cheese and "French" fries cooked in hydrogenated, trans-fatty acids, pastries high in sugar and fat content, and, of course, sodas rich with sugar all gathered together to make us fat. A typical McDonalds "Quarter-Pounder with Cheese" itself contains 510 calories and includes about 12 grams of saturated fat, over 1,000 milligrams of sodium, 90 milligrams of cholesterol and 40 grams of carbohydrates. Add to this another 130 calories for a soda and about 380 calories for a medium serving of "French" fries yields a total of more than 1,000 calories. But, McDonald's actually doesn't lead the pack. In fact, it really depends upon precisely what is eaten at the popular fast food chains that matters. A similar meal at either Wendy's or Burger King yields about the same number of calories as that of McDonalds.

Prior to the fast food culture and one that still prevails to a small extent today was the so called "TV Dinner" culture. TV dinners are well-balanced meals prepared and pre-frozen for ease of cooking and dispensation from a conventional, convection or microwave oven. Although TV dinners were generally prepared with all of the necessary food groups, most such meals were prepared from processed foods rich in carbohydrates and saturated fats, all seasoned heavily for taste, especially with sodium. A typical TV dinner contains far fewer calories, however, than something one could obtain at a typical fast-food restaurant. Most TV dinners consist of about 300-500 calories each; but, the fact that they are processed with preservatives and contain high concentrations of sodium tends to balance the scale.

3. The Gender Culture

An important observation in regard to the rates of obesity is that in virtually every race or ethnic classification, the rate of obesity among females is always higher than among males. This does not mean, of course, that females have less self-control than males; however, part of the reason may relate in fact to measures of control. In many cultures of the world, females are regarded with much less status than males. In fact, it was only until the turn of 20th century that females in the United States began to assert themselves and achieve greater equality with males. But prior to that, the role of females had always been relegated to menial and far less aggressive activities than that of males. Males were always the hunters and gatherers, while females were the caretakers and nurturers. By contrast to the active-aggressive lifestyles led by most males, females had always been sustained into a passive-aggressive or sedentary lifestyle.

Even in modern times, the role of females is still much less active, in general, than that of the average male. For example, it is rare to find females working in construction jobs or jobs requiring heavy lifting, pushing and pulling. Up until recently, the role of females even in the military services was relegated almost exclusively to support activities and very few, if any, were trained for and/or served in combat roles. Most females in the work force take jobs that are administrative in general. After all, females are still considered the weaker gender in terms of their physical characteristics. Nevertheless, this distinction is biologically predisposed to making women genetically more likely to become obese strictly by the nature of their sex.

C. Obesity: A World Pandemic

As China and Russia became more westernized, this of course exacerbated the obesity problem almost exclusively by the inclusion of the massive populations of these nations into the world obesity statistical rolls. Indeed, prior to the 20th century obesity was rare and its prevalence only notable in developing nations. By 2008, however, almost 10% of the world's population or about 400 million adults, most of them female and the elderly are considered obese and more than 1 billion are considered overweight. In fact, the World Health Organization (WHO) now considers obesity a *pandemic*. Unlike the term *epidemic*, which is used to describe a health condition or disease that spreads over a large localized region, a pandemic is one that has worldwide significance.

The most notable reason for the increased rate and proliferation of obesity, according to the World Health Organization, is an increased consumption of more energy dense foods, nutrition-poor foods and foods high in saturated fats and sugar. The availability and variety of such foods worldwide through international trade and complex distribution systems is only part of the reason for this trend. Rapid urbanization and modernization are partly to blame in that these factors have contributed to a decrease in human activity levels. In the Third-World cultures, lack of education about the content and nutritional value of certain foods has contributed significantly to the high rates of obesity therein.

Another factor that may be contributing to global obesity is that, although war continues to prevail in many countries, it is not on the scale experienced during World War I and World War II. Consequently, world trade is not impeded by naval blockades, submarine attacks and national isolation. War contributes invariably to rationing, famine and a general interruption of the global distribution and trade systems. Moreover, the massive build-up of military infrastructure from large-scale wars draws resources significantly away from civilian population centers leaving the latter much to their own survival. Today, wars are mere conflicts and are isolated to specific regions or countries. Weapons of war have become so sophisticated that the mere notion of another world war conjures fears of planetary destruction and human extinction.

D. Childhood Obesity

Television and computers have been especially implicated in the rapid onset of childhood obesity. This has been complicated by the reactionary change in defensive behaviors resulting from media coverage of terrorism and crime, most notably crimes against children. Up until as late as the 1980's it was not uncommon to see children playing in the streets, at playgrounds and around the neighborhood for hours each day. Children played vigorously and largely unsupervised. But, the advent of television and computer internet services made it possible to convey detailed news events on a scale never before experienced, even during the radio days of the early 1900's. While many believe that the per capita rate of crime has really not changed throughout history, what has changed is society's cognitive awareness of crime from its media coverage. Media coverage has somehow sewn the unintended seed of fear and anxiety especially among parents for their children. Consequently, children are now a highly protected species who rarely go out to play except under close supervision and at organized events.

1. Prisoners of Technology

More than ever before, children must stay home, at a day care center or in school. At home, the only activities readily available to fulfill the restless nature of children are television and computer video games. Children have thus become much less active and certainly much more prone to becoming obese. This trend is further complicated by the fact many schools no longer mandate active recess periods and physical education curriculums. Moreover, because children must now be carefully supervised when engaged in outdoor activities, this requires time from parents that has now become a veritable luxury.

The statistics related to childhood obesity are alarming and correlate directly to the advent of television and computer technology. According to the Centers for Disease Control and the U.S. Department of Health and Human Services, more than 13% of children and adolescents in the United States are considered obese. More alarming is that the rate of obesity among children and adolescents had almost doubled between 1950 and 1980, the period during which television began to permeate society. But, since 1980, about the time when personal computers were introduced, the rate of obesity among children and adolescents had more than tripled.

An even more alarming development is that peer pressure is no longer a factor in helping to control childhood obesity. Until recently, very few children were obese and thus were usually the targets of harassment and railing from peers. This often led to corrective behavior. Today, there are so many obese children that they tend to blend in and their conditions taken for granted. Although many children eventually grow out of their obese state many sustain the behavior that resulted in their obese state in the first place throughout their adult lives. Even though children are young and potentially active enough to resolve their weight problem, the collateral health consequences of this condition even for a short duration can be dangerous and chronic.

Childhood obesity is more than just a social problem. For example children are much more likely to develop risk factors for cardiovascular disease than adults. These include hypertension, high levels of blood cholesterol and all of the precursors to Type II diabetes, including insulin resistance. Obese children are also more likely than children of normal weight to become obese as adults. Obese children are also more inclined to develop bone and joint problems, sleep apnea and many of the psychosocial problems associated with obesity such as lack of self-esteem, potential drug and alcohol abuse and suicidal tendencies.

2. Task Force on Childhood Obesity

Childhood obesity, especially in the United States, has become so prevalent that in 2009, an ambitious campaign was launched by First Lady Michelle Obama called "Let's Move". The campaign resulted in the formation by President Barack Obama of the Task Force on Childhood Obesity. This task force included the U.S. Department of Education, USDA, the U.S. Department of the Interior, the U.S. Department of Health and Human Services and several other agencies. The purpose of the campaign was to evaluate the current state and causes of childhood obesity and to develop programs to combat the problem. Such programs would include the restoration of mandatory physical education activities in schools, strict adherence by public school food services departments to proper dietary and nutritional standards and broad programs of health education which expressly teach the dangers of obesity.

The Obama Campaign included many new federal directives aimed at changing the health patterns of children. The Food and Drug Administration was directed, for example, to enhance and enforce food labeling standards by food manufacturers and distributors. Major media campaigns were launched, targeting especially the parents to educate them on the dangers of childhood obesity and the many ways in which the condition can be managed and resolved. The campaign also resulted in the reauthorization of the Child Nutrition Act of 2004 which regulated the content and quality of foods served in schools. The act covers many collateral school funding programs for meals served in public schools, including the National School Breakfast Program and the National School Lunch Program. It called for the expansion of the National Food and Nutrition Service and its Fresh Fruit and Vegetable Program and substantially improved the nutritional standards by which foods must be processed, prepared and served in public schools.

One of the most significant changes brought about by the Let's Move campaign is the restoration of mandatory physical education programs in public schools. For years prior to 1980, most public schools required all students to enroll into a physical education program and to engage in periodic rest and recreational activities in school. Student injuries and resulting civil litigation led to a rapid waning of these programs until most schools did not offer them at all or simply offered physical education as an elective. Some schools even eliminated organized sports activities such as football and basketball to avoid the possibility of civil litigation. Part of the intent of the Let's Move campaign is to initiate tort reform that would hold public schools harmless from litigation for non-negligent causes of action. Many public schools will be required to again provide mandatory physical education programs, but will be empowered to design their programs for maximum safety. Among the safety standards proposed by the new standards will be school health program and enrollment pre-requisite that would require students to obtain basic health physicals, such physicals performed to detect underlying conditions that may preclude students from engaging in vigorous physical exercise programs.

E. Chapter Summary

As of 2008 more than one billion people worldwide are considered overweight and more than a third of these are considered obese or morbidly obese. Although the problem of obesity is prevalent most in the industrialized, developed nations of the world it is becoming more of a problem even in the Third-World cultures. Although there are wide deviations in the prevalence and rate of obesity across race and ethnic lines, this appears to be the result of behaviors associated with poverty and lack of education. Political suppression resulting in lack of industrialization, urbanization and international trade may have helped to prevent the onset of obesity from food rationing and nutritional restrictions in countries such as China and Russia. Since these countries have become more westernized their prevalence and rate of obesity has increased at an alarming rate. Childhood obesity has become a growing problem given to the advent of technology, an increase in defensive behaviors resulting from crimes against children and a decline in emphasis on physical activity in public schools. To combat this development First Lady Michelle Obama launched her Let's Move campaign which led to the formation of President Barack Obama's Task Force of Childhood Obesity.

Key Points:

1. Obesity is a worldwide pandemic
2. Obesity is probably not caused by a difference in race and ethnicity but rather by poverty and lack of education across racial classifications
3. The rate and prevalence of obesity may have been delayed in certain countries by political suppression
4. The Fast Food culture has contributed significantly to obesity worldwide
5. Childhood obesity may be the result of technology such as television and personal computers
6. The Task Force on Childhood Obesity was organized to increase education and awareness of the dangers of childhood obesity and to develop programs to resolve this health issue

7. The Childhood Nutrition Act of 2004 was reauthorized as a result of First Lady Michelle Obama's Let's Move campaign to eliminate childhood obesity

Chapter 7—*the Economics of Obesity*

When we explored the many health risks and dangers associated with obesity in **Chapter 4**, the reader may have intuitively reasoned how that must influence the cost of health care. In fact, obesity is now one of the main reasons why health care costs are increasing, especially in the United States. In 2009, health care costs rose to $147 billion to make up almost 16% of the Gross Domestic Product (GDP). It is estimated that by 2018 medical costs associated with obesity will rise to about $344 billion or about 22% of the GDP. This is alarming considering that the average cost of healthcare as a percent of the GDP among developed nations of the world is only about 8.4%. These statistics are particularly disconcerting considering that affordable health care is becoming much less accessible. Meanwhile, health insurance rates are rising beyond the point at which many Americans can even afford to carry it. This means that many more uninsured Americans will clutter hospital emergency rooms and thus help to further increase health care costs, including higher health insurance rates and charges by health care providers.

The insidious formula for a nationwide and eventually perhaps, even a worldwide health care cost disaster is fundamentally simple. Obesity leads to many major illnesses which require medical intervention. The average obese individual, in fact, will cost about 42% more in healthcare delivery services than an individual of normal weight according to the American Public Health Association. Not only does obesity result in compelling medical costs, but also in costs associated with preventive and interventional medicine. Between 2000 and 2009 more than $18 billion was spent by obese consumers for cosmetic intervention, including tummy tucks, bariatric surgery and liposuction.

Despite the rising cost of healthcare as a consequence of obesity, it's really a double-edged sword when one considers the enormous amount spent on advertising and food promotions that contribute to obesity. Food promotions, including TV commercials and billboard advertising of delectable foods and even TV cooking programs tend to influence the onset of obesity. At the same time, the litany of dietary supplements, diet programs and diet fads and similar inducements make up a multi-billion dollar industry which both fosters and capitalizes upon obese consumers. Corporations that market diet programs want their customers to be fat just as auto repair shops want cars to break down. It's all about economics; and, that these programs are aimed to eliminate obesity altogether is sheer nonsense.

A. Obesity and Healthcare Costs

The burden of obesity upon the health care industry is alarming at best. In fact, healthcare costs associated with obesity are almost twice that of those related to smoking and three times that of those related to alcohol and drug abuse. The most significant costs related to obesity are for the treatment of obesity-related illness such as Type II diabetes, elevated cholesterol, hypertension and cardiovascular disease. Private health insurance spending on illnesses related to obesity has increased more than ten times since 1987 according to a 15-year study conducted by Emory University under the direction of Kenneth Thorpe. In fact, from 1987 to 2002 the amount spent by employers and privately insured families on obesity-related illnesses rose from about 2% to almost 12%. As of 2010, the figure is now 18% according to the Centers for Disease Control (CDC) in Atlanta, Georgia.

Not only does the burden of obesity affect healthcare costs directly, it is also having a deleterious influence upon nationwide productivity. Because obese individuals tend to spend more time on visits to a doctor for obesity-related illness, this has resulted in a significant increase in employee absenteeism. Work-related injuries associated with obesity are also being blamed for the rising cost of healthcare. In fact, obese individuals are more likely to be injured in the work place than those of normal weight. The unintended consequence of absenteeism and work-related injuries is a closer scrutiny by employers in their hiring practices. Although it is very likely discriminatory to base hiring practices upon one's health, weight is not identified among the protective covenants of the Civil Rights Act of 1964. Consequently, employers are finding many creative ways to avoid hiring obese individuals.

Regardless of what employers may do to avoid hiring obese individuals, with more than 65% of the United States population considered as being overweight, the odds are against them. Indeed, as more and more obese individuals permeate the work force, the consequential reduction in productivity will mean that more work must be done to produce the same goods and services. Employers faced with this reality will take the usual defensive measures and pass the additional cost of productivity on to the consumer. So, now you not only have an increase in healthcare costs related to obesity but also the general rate of inflation associated with reduced productivity and increased absenteeism in the work force. As the rate of inflation increases so too will the demand for higher pay. Employers faced with this reality will likely react by reducing their work force thus contributing to an increase in the rate of unemployment. Higher unemployment means that many more individuals will likely be uninsured and consequently impose yet another burden upon the cost of healthcare. It is indeed a precarious and self-destructive cycle.

Although many believe that obesity is economically burdensome, there is another side to this coin. Indeed, while obese individuals may burden the healthcare system through increased access for obesity-related medical conditions, these same individuals, by the very nature of their conditions, are less likely to live long lives. Many of the diseases and conditions which are derived from being obese, are themselves life threatening and can thus significantly reduce life expectancy, especially among those over the age of 50 years.

1. Socialized Healthcare

Obesity-related health care costs are taking their toll upon an already burgeoning problem plaguing the United States which is among the few nations of the world that has not yet adopted a universal, socialized healthcare delivery system. If the rate of obesity continues to increase as it has in the past three decades, it may become the ultimate catalyst for the creation of a universal healthcare delivery system or a system of socialized, government-regulated medicine. With universal healthcare, the party will be essentially over, not only for healthcare providers, but also for healthcare consumers. Healthcare providers will see a dramatic decrease in their incomes while healthcare consumers may face long lines and healthcare rationing. Under a socialized healthcare system, healthcare consumers will likely be required to enroll in preventive health programs just to obtain affordable healthcare coverage.

Socialized medicine in the United States is among the most controversial issues of modern times because many believe that such as system will almost invariably eliminate choice and in some way regulate the lifestyles of healthcare consumers. Indeed, if the government becomes burdened with the responsibility of insuring all Americans, it will likely develop programs and policies to mitigate healthcare costs. They may require that all Americans obtain a physical examination at least once each year. Policies may be established requiring healthcare providers to strictly enforce preventive health protocols upon their patients. Such protocols may include strict diets and exercise regiments, abstention from smoking and alcohol consumption. Even employers will not escape the burdens of such a system. Employers under socialized healthcare will likely be required to provide routine exercise and recreational activities for employees whose job responsibilities are sedentary or clerical in nature.

If the socialized healthcare system is constructed fairly, it would require limiting the amount earned by healthcare providers, including physicians, allied health professionals, pharmaceutical companies, medical equipment and supply manufacturers and so on. The reason for this is that socialized healthcare system will be subsidized by state and federal income taxes. Consequently, on one hand, the average American will likely be paying higher taxes while on the other hand fewer individuals will likely choose healthcare as a career profession. Meanwhile, because all individuals under a socialized healthcare delivery system will be able to affordably access healthcare services, they will likely do so more regularly. This could further burden the system through increased waiting lines, limited physician visitations and a general rationing of care. Consequently, many Americans may not obtain the services they need.

The preceding discussion may seem like the theme of a classic horror film, but as the debate rages over socialized medicine, Americans continue to become overweight and healthcare costs continue to rise. Indeed, at some point, the bubble must burst. As healthcare costs rise beyond the point that even minor treatments for cuts and abrasions can lead to personal bankruptcy, the system itself will implode. In fact, as of the publication of this book, more than half of all personal bankruptcies filed in the United States were the result of healthcare costs, especially those for out-of-pocket expenses to finance catastrophic illnesses or injuries. More than two million Americans were among those filing for bankruptcy as a direct result of the burden of healthcare costs. Even more alarming than this is that more than two-thirds of those filing medical bankruptcy were insured. As more and more Americans file for bankruptcy in response to the rising cost of healthcare, the system will continue pass these costs on to those who can afford to pay them until the latter too will feel the pinch. As the medical cost-related bankruptcy rate continues it will eventually bankrupt the healthcare delivery system itself.

Many believe that the only effective way in which to create an equitable and successful universal healthcare system is to eliminate the for-profit motive of the healthcare industry. Indeed, most of the entities that make up the healthcare industry, including private, investor owned hospitals, pharmaceutical companies, private health insurance companies, healthcare equipment, supplies and services companies, physicians and private clinics are all in the business of making a profit. For-profit companies will usually act in the best interest of their shareholders or owners. Critics of a non-profit, universal healthcare system argue that the absence of a profit motive will inhibit industry innovation and growth. Still others believe that, in addition to the elimination of the profit motive, there should also be an elimination or overhaul of the congressional lobby system, especially those involving healthcare corporate interests. Critics of the congressional lobby system believe it to be a breeding ground for corruption and "favored nation" policies. Many argue that congressional lobbies favor powerful financial interests often at the expense of the smaller or less effective ones, as well as the average healthcare consumer. Advocates of the congressional lobby system argue that it is often the only way to address the attention of legislators on various issues that may not otherwise interest them.

Another major barrier to the successful creation of a universal healthcare system is frivolous and unreasonably costly civil litigation. Although litigation tends to help police incompetency among healthcare providers, it tends to also be a breeding ground for corruption. Indeed, many civil cases result in unreasonably high settlements for largely unnecessary or frivolous law suits. These settlements are passed onto healthcare providers in higher malpractice premiums which in turn lead to defensive behaviors by healthcare providers. But although this would tend to improve healthcare quality, it also increases healthcare costs to the patients in higher health insurance premiums. Many believe that tort reform is necessary to combat corruptive practices in civil litigation. Such reforms should include pre-litigation hearings to evaluate case validity and feasibility, limits on settlements paid as well as limits on attorneys fees derived from such settlements. The major barrier to tort reform legislation is that most of the legislators are themselves attorneys.

2. Health Insurance and Managed Care

The last frontier of protection against catastrophic loss related to illness or injury is health insurance. Indeed, health insurance has long been a shelter of financial catastrophe against rising healthcare costs. But, recently, even health insurance companies are beginning to posture themselves against rising healthcare costs. In addition to having almost tripled medical premiums in the past thirty years, health insurance companies have also begun increasing their deductibles and co-pay requirements. More disconcerting is that many services formerly covered by health insurance have been dropped, especially those for elective and preventive healthcare. While it may be logical to eliminate insurance for elective-cosmetic surgery, it has now become a trend among insurance companies to eliminate coverage for health physicals, medical screening exams and routine x-rays, mammograms and other early detection measures.

Even though health care costs appear to be rising because of increased consumer demand, there are those who believe that the industry is equally to blame. For example, although the insurance companies complain about rising health care costs, health care insurance is still very big business. To illustrate a case in point, the average amount spent per person per year for health care is about $6,500. Now, the average health insurance premiums per year for covered individuals total about $450 per month per person or about $5,400 per year. This amount carries an average deductible of about $500 per year plus at least 20% for the co-pay (shared out-of-pocket) amount. So let's add this up! The average person pays $5,400 for health insurance, but accesses $6,500 worth of health care services, $500 of which is paid up front for the deductible requirement plus another 20% of the $6,000 balance or $1,200. Consequently, the average person pays a total of $1,200 + $500 + $5,400 = $7,100 for $6,500 worth of healthcare. But, this is only for covered health care services. Suppose that, of the $6,500, about $1,000 is for services not covered by the health insurance policy. This raises the total out-of-pocket expense to the average consumer to $8,100 per year for $6,500 worth of healthcare services.

An interesting paradox that now prevails with regard to health insurance is that an "ounce of prevention" is no longer worth "a pound of cure". A case in point can be made with a typical home owner's insurance policy. Most companies that underwrite such policies do not pay the cost to remove a tree even if it has the potential of crashing through the roof of one's home. In this case, if the tree does indeed damage the home, the insurance company has essentially foregone $1,000 to remove the tree before it falls in favor of $20,000 to finance repairs on the home. Ironically, these repairs also include removal of the fallen tree. Insurance companies argue, however, that coverage for prevention would actually tend to increase the cost of insurance because more individuals would use the coverage, for example, to remove trees regardless of whether or not they could fall on one's home. In the case of healthcare coverage, the cost to provide breast cancer screens twice each year for the life of 100 insured individuals, for example, may actually exceed the cost of treating breast cancer for the 12 among these who are statistically likely to develop the disease.

Given the preceding paradox in regard to healthcare insurance coverage, imagine paying the cost of obesity clinics, dietary supplements and weight loss programs for the number of Americans who are considered obese. This would likely burden the insurance companies far beyond their ability to cover the more critical healthcare issues. The answer then may be to place the burden of prevention upon the healthcare provider. Instead of relying upon the insurance consumer to stay healthy, make it the responsibility of the physician. This rather interesting notion had actually given rise to an innovative and indeed, very unique method by which health insurance coverage would be administered—*Managed Care*. But, as we shall discover, Managed Care was conceived, not necessarily to improve preventive medicine, but primarily to control the cost of providing insurance coverage—to increase profitability among health insurance companies.

Managed care was originally conceived as an alternative to the traditional indemnity insurance plans. Under the latter plans, healthcare providers were reimbursed for services rendered. Even if providers increased their charges for services, as well as the intensity of services provided, they would be reimbursed likewise. Unfortunately, viewing this as rather a pot of gold, many providers took advantage of the system by performing unnecessary and superfluous services as a means of increasing their personal earnings. As this type of fraudulent activity began to permeate the healthcare industry, it threatened to bankrupt the health insurance companies. It also contributed to an increase in healthcare costs, especially from higher premiums.

Contrary to the traditional indemnity plans, with a typical managed care system, health insurance coverage is provided through an integrated delivery system in which physicians and hospitals network to manage a specific number of covered lives for a fixed periodic reimbursement rate. Two models that have emerged from the network delivery concept are the HMO (Health Maintenance Organization) and the PPO (Preferred Provider Organization). With a PPO, the health insurance company contracts with specific healthcare providers known as "preferred providers" to care for all the patients that are enrolled in the plan. Patients enrolled in a PPO can choose any physician they desire as long as the physician is part of the network. Otherwise, they must pay additional out-of-pocket expenses. The HMO is considerably more restrictive than the PPO in that, instead of reimbursing physicians under a fixed-rate payment contract, it employs a limited number of primary care physicians who are specifically assigned to care for a certain number of patients for a specified salary. The patients, in this case, have no choice of provider and must be seen by the physician to whom they are assigned.

The way in which the typical managed care system works is that each provider is reimbursed a pre-negotiated, contract amount per insured or covered enrollee each month regardless of the number of patients actually seen. This method is commonly referred as *capitation.* For example, suppose Dr. Jones is a network provider for 100 covered patients. The insurance company contracts with Dr. Jones, to pay him, for example, $1,500 per covered life for a total of $125,000 per month, regardless of the number of patients seen. This $1,500 per covered life is expected to pay all of Dr. Jones costs, including his salary, for the care of any of the patients he treats who are specifically enrolled in the plan. Suppose now that Dr. Jones sees 70 patients per month at an average cost of about $1,600 each. This equates to $120,000 per month leaving Dr. Jones a profit of $5,000 or about $60,000 per year. If the average cost of each of the 70 patients seen was instead $1,900 per month, Dr. Jones would incur a loss of $8,000 or about $96,000 per year.

The preceding example should make it clear that managed care reimbursement can offer inducements to physicians that can play the system effectively. To do so, these physicians must insure that the cost to care for each such patient does not exceed the capitation payment amount. The advantage of this type of payment system is that physicians will attempt to do their best to keep their patients healthy. This may include free health screenings and fewer unnecessary services and procedures. It may also mean fewer prescriptions and prescriptions of generic instead of brand-name drugs. The disadvantage of this approach is that healthcare quality may decline as a consequence of rationing. Physicians desiring to maximize profits may do so at the patient's expense. Fortunately, the guiding-hand function of consequence may prevail against physicians who ration their services too much. In this instance, their patients' health may decline to the point that more intense and costly services would be required in the long run. It may also result in civil litigation against the physician.

The capitation payment system offers substantial opportunities for reducing, regulating or controlling healthcare costs simply by its inherent guiding-hand nature. Physicians with enrolled patients who are overweight or obese will likely enforce clinical measures to manage the problem in order to avoid the cost of obesity-related illnesses and a resulting higher intensity and cost of healthcare services in the long run. On the other hand, many physicians may demand higher rates of capitation for obese patients than for patients of normal weight. This notion brings us to another one of the many reasons why healthcare costs are rising. Owing to the higher costs associated with managing obese patients, insurance companies have been compelled to raise their rates in order to provide reasonable capitation payments to providers. Moreover, physicians can still increase the fees that they charge in order to recover any of their capitation losses from the patient's co-payment requirement and for services not covered by the patient's insurance plan.

The problem of higher insurance rates brings us back to the basics of healthcare economics. Indeed, many of the large and medium sized employers offer health insurance as a benefit to their employees. These employers can obtain substantial discounts for what are known as group health insurance plans. The more lives that are covered by a typical group health plan, the lower the rate per covered life. But as healthcare costs have continued to rise over the past 30 years, many employers, especially those having fewer than 50 employees have dropped their benefit coverage altogether. Moreover, many of the larger companies no longer offer family coverage for their employees. Instead, their employees are given the option of covering family members at the lower group rate. Those companies that have sustained their employee health benefits have passed the additional cost of coverage onto their customers.

B. Obesity and the Industrial Complex

When we contemplate the enormous impact upon healthcare costs that obesity appears to impose, it is quite tempting and often compelling to acquire emotions of disdain over this problem. To be fair, however, we must apportion the blame by giving due consideration to all of the many predispositions to obesity. We must also contend with the possibility that the solution to obesity is being economically suppressed. By this, I mean that the problem of obesity is actually a multibillion dollar industry. While obesity may be causing substantial increases in healthcare costs, it is simultaneously feeding the healthcare industry which must allocate more resources to manage the problem—not obesity itself, but the health problems that result from being obese.

Imagine what would happen if, in one day, a cure was found for all forms of cancer. Within a very short period of time, the administration of a simple vaccine would eliminate the disease altogether. Meanwhile, the pharmaceutical companies would lose billions of dollars in revenues from drugs used in chemotherapy. Providers specializing in cancer treatment and care such as oncologists and radiation therapists would have to change careers overnight. Cancer surgery would be completely eliminated. Hospitals and nursing homes would also lose billions in revenue from their loss of convalescing cancer patients. The economic impact goes even further considering that the massive loss in healthcare revenues would impose a ripple effect that would include massive layoffs, business foreclosures and possibly even a stock market crash. This would lead to an increase in the unemployment rate and a corresponding reduction in consumer spending and the downward spiral would continue.

In recent times, we have all seen how the insolvency of large industrial complexes can have disastrous economic consequences. In fact, during the George Bush and Barack Obama presidencies, the U.S. government spent billions of dollars in so called "bail-outs" of large automobile and insurance companies as well as large banking institutions just to avoid the far-reaching economic adversities the failure of these industries would impose upon society in general. Indeed, change is often necessary in order to achieve growth and prosperity, but it must come insidiously and gradually to avoid a shock to the system. So, even though everything conceivable must be done to solve the obesity problem there must be a commitment to do so by those who now profit from it.

C. Obesity in the Market Place

Imagine that you are an American, pre-colonial homemaker. There are no refrigerators and cooking is very likely done in a cast-iron skillet over a wood fire. It is early dawn and your family wants some breakfast, so you go out to your own chicken coup if you're lucky to have one and gather some eggs. You would then rustle up some flour you may have ground yourself to make biscuits. You have a baby and some toddlers that need milk, so you go out to the barn and milk one of your cows. By the time you gather everything needed for breakfast, it has already taken perhaps a couple of hours or so. Then you cook, not just for yourself, but for everyone in the family. Meanwhile, your husband is very likely plowing the field or out hunting for lunch and dinner. The latter two meals are even more challenging, especially if you want meat. If you want chicken, well … you or your husband would have to go out, butcher it, pluck it then put it on a spit over the fire. Otherwise, if your husband hunted some squirrels, he would have to skin them and you can imagine the rest.

The preceding scenario describes an extremely laborious daily routine for preparing meals. The work involved, in this case, would probably require most, if not all the activity calories one would consume from the meal itself. By contrast to the rigorous meal preparations of the past, now we can simply drive to the local grocer and, once there, be confronted with so much variety and choice that we could spend hours just in evaluating a few product lines. Then there are the numerous sales, specials and give-away samples, all engineered to get us to buy the products whether we need them or not. In fact, food distribution companies spend millions of dollars each year just in their product promotions, painstakingly making their products appear appetizing and delectable in order to induce maximum sales.

Adding convenience of access to the variety and availability of food, we now have a formula for self-destructive behavior beyond anything experienced in history. It's not just at the local grocer where we're confronted with the temptations of food. There is also a litany of television commercials about food, most of which are aired at precisely the times during which we would likely want to dine. Then there are the newspaper ads, coupled with hundreds of coupons to reinforce our appetite for food. But commercials and newspaper advertising are simply not enough. Now we can watch dozens of television programs featuring world renowned chefs, most of whom are also obese or overweight, all showing us the many creative and clever ways to tease our taste buds.

1. Food Marketing and Advertising Target Children

Although newspapers and magazines have been traditionally used by food distribution companies to advertise their products, the electronic media, especially television and the internet are now the primary sources of advertising. A remarkable finding with respect to television advertising it that it appears to target children more readily than it does adults. The reason for this is that children watch television more frequently and for longer periods of time than adults. But, even more pervasive is the proliferation of food advertising on the internet. This is based also upon to the notion that children, more so than adults, will use a computer for casual and frivolous pursuit. While advertising food products to children may seem rather innocuous, it is illusive and provocative at best. Indeed, advertising to children focuses, not upon sound nutritional practice, but almost solely upon taste. In other words, for advertisers, it's not important that children eat what's right but rather what they like, such as sweats like cookies, candy and soda and foods high in saturated fats such as pizza, hamburgers, cheeseburgers, etc.

The children of today clearly live in a media-saturated environment and, because of their youthful age, are easily influenced by the advertising culture without really understanding its significance. Because children watch a lot of television, this then is the largest single source of advertising next to the internet. In fact, more than 75% of the advertising budgets of most U.S. food manufacturers and distributors are allocated for television content. With the fast-food restaurant industry, television advertising is even higher, making up a whopping the 95% of the advertising budgets of the major fast-food chains such as McDonalds and Kentucky Fried Chicken. So saturated is television with media advertising that the average child may view up to 40,000 commercials each year. Every five minutes that a child watches television, he/she is exposed to at least one food-related commercial and may view up to three hours of food-related commercials each week. With this in mind, it's a small wonder why childhood obesity is so high.

Food-related advertising to children is certainly not confined to television and the internet. In fact, this media blitz has actually begun to transcend into the nation's public schools. In many public schools throughout the U.S. students can purchase soft drinks and snacks from vending machines and name-brand, fast-food products from the cafeteria. The reason school marketing of food is successful is that the food manufacturers and distributors offer lucrative contract incentives to the school districts such as donated equipment and sharing of their percentage of sales and/or profits. In some cases, even teachers are offered personal incentives to advertise the products of certain food vendors. They do so with t-shirt logos and magnetic ads on their cars and are paid educational stipends or school supply coupons.

The marketing and advertising of food products to children has been deemed quite successful based upon numerous studies. Such studies showed that children exposed to advertising were much more likely to choose advertised food products than children who were not exposed. Although most children do not have the resources to simply go out and purchase what they see in advertisements, studies have shown that they have a significant influence upon their parents' shopping habits. Children will make numerous attempts to convince parents to buy the food products they want and, in most cases, the parents will concede. Even the parents themselves can be influenced by food advertisements specifically targeting children. Marketing engineers devise clever advertising schemes that associate adult food products with products that children would likely consume. An example of this is advertising by fast-food restaurants at which children can eat free if one or more parents purchase a meal.

The massive onslaught of media advertising to children has led to sweeping legislative controls on advertising, as well as increased scrutiny by the Federal Communications Commission and Federal Trade Commission. The advertising industry itself maintains its own non-profit regulatory agency known as the Children's Advertising Review Unit (CARU); but, the CARU has very little power or authority and can only suggest advertising policy to private, independent corporations. Even though many rules had been established to regulate advertising to children since 1970, powerful lobby interests kept it largely anemic. It wasn't until 1980 that congress passed the Children's Advertising Act (CAA) as a consequence of intense public pressure. The CAA prohibited certain types of advertising to children, but more importantly, limited the amount the amount of commercial time related to food advertising during children's programming, especially on weekends.

2. Marketing Nutrition and Health

Yet another pervasive practice among advertisers is the label food products with deceptive claims of food content and nutritional value. Indeed, as federal controls on food processing and labeling become stricter, advertisers are finding more and more clever ways in which to overcome this trend. After all, the objective of advertising is sell a given product, and it is very likely much easier to sell a cheeseburger than it is to sell a can of spinach. It gets even more subtle when you factor in the grower consumer scrutiny of food values such as the number of calories per serving, proportion per serving of transfatty acids, saturated fats, sugar and sodium. As a consequence of federal labeling standards and the proliferation of health-related advertising, the lay consumer is becoming more educated on matters of nutrition and health. Despite, this however, the high rate of obesity prevails more than likely because the actual content of food really hasn't changed much. Moreover, no matter what the labels may suggest or whatever warnings may be evident from the distribution of various components of food, it is very difficult to change one's eating habits strictly on the basis of nutritional value.

Most analysts readily agree that food labeling has done little if anything to change the habits of food shoppers. It's sort of like reading the warning labels on a pack of cigarettes. If you are a habitual smoker, such labels will likely be ignored. With food labeling, the problem is not so much the information on the labels, but the time and effort it would take to evaluate and, for that matter, even to carefully measure the content of various ingredients. Realistically, it would take hours perhaps to shop for a week's worth of groceries if each product purchased is carefully evaluated for nutritional content and value. Then there is also the *elasticity of demand*. Elasticity of demand refers to how much a typical consumer is willing alter his/her demand for certain products based upon various factors such a price, brand loyalty, health reasons, taste, marketing influence, etc. An example would be whether or not someone would begin buying turkey burgers instead of beef burgers to reduce the consumption of fat. If there is absolutely nothing that would influence a change in demand for beef burgers, then the consumer preference for this product would be inelastic. Otherwise, if someone is easily influenced to change from beef burgers to turkey burgers then the demand for beef burgers would be elastic.

The elasticity of demand is particularly critical in the battle against obesity since there are now numerous healthy substitutes for various food products. Whole milk products can now be replaced with skim milk or 2% milk and cheeses made from whole milk can now be substituted for those made with skim milk. There is also a great variety of substitution in the beverage market with diet sodas and light beers and many brand-name products are now available in both regular and diet varieties. Of course, any consumer demand for these substitutes is indeed dependent upon their elasticity. After all, many diet or low-fat substitutes for certain food products are not necessarily as appetizing as those in their traditional state. It took many years, for example, to alter the eating habits of consumers accustomed to frying foods in lard instead of vegetable oil or shortening almost invariably because of the perceived difference in taste. In similar fashion, products high in sodium content always seem to taste better than those made with salt substitutes or no salt at all. In fact, many consumers who buy low-sodium food products will go home and cook them then sprinkle salt on them anyway. So what's the point of even buying the product? Indeed, most dietary substitutes actually cost more than the traditional food products because of the specialized processing methods required to produce them.

The other problem with dietary substitutes is that they often leave us hungry for more; hence, instead of helping to resolve the problem of obesity, they may actually worsen it. Some dietary products are actually sold with less of one ingredient, but more of another in order to make up for their loss of taste from the way in which they are processed. Many products low in saturated or transfats are given higher doses of sodium or monosodium glutamate, again to overcome diminished taste. Low fat and skim milk products are given a much higher dose of sugar to help in diminishing their watery taste. Skim milk also includes certain chemicals to thicken it to the consistency of whole milk.

D. Chapter Summary

As a consequence of the alarming increase in the number of overweight and obese individuals, healthcare costs associated with managing the health consequences of these conditions are increasing also. Presently, about 16% of the Gross Domestic Product (GNP) or about $147 million is spend for healthcare costs related to obesity. The average obese individual spends about 42% more for health care than an individual of normal weight. Even though health care costs related to obesity are increasing at an alarming rate, the fact that it has become a self-sustaining, multibillion dollar industry

Key Points:

1. Health care costs related to obesity make up about16% of the GDP
2. The average obese individual will spend 42% more in health care than a person of normal weight
3. The health insurance, pharmaceutical and other allied health industries are profiting from obesity
4. Marketing and advertising of food products specifically target children
5. Food labeling standards have not had a significant impact on consumer spending

Section III

How to Manage Obesity

Chapter 8—*Diet and Exercise*

The two most common treatments for obesity are diet and exercise. While these may seem the logical approach to managing the problem, they come with several little known caveats. Indeed, the term diet has many different meanings and exercise comes in many different forms. Some diets may involve a reduction in the amount of food consumed per day, but others may result in an increase in the total consumption of food but a decrease in the caloric value of such foods. In either case, the objective is to reduce the total number of calories consumed per day. At the same time, it is necessary to increase the human metabolic rate through some form of exercise. The reason for this is that when the body consumes fewer calories it will venture into starvation mode and thus begin to automatically lower its metabolic rate. Remember that energy calories are required just to digest foods. This is called thermic metabolism. So, as fewer calories are consumed, thermic metabolism will actually decline. At the same time, when a person exercises, this increases activity metabolism which in turn will tend to increase appetite. Appetite is conjured by the body when it demands more calories for energy.

An appropriate analogy to describe the management of obesity through diet and exercise is perhaps that it's like "…a salmon swimming upstream". Indeed, diet and exercise are usually meted with several countervailing forces. The most significant of these is perseverance. One must have the sustained will to maintain a normal weight in order, not only to lose weight, but also, and probably more importantly, to keep it off. But the force that rages against perseverance is physics. As the body ages, more work is required to maintain a normal body mass; and, the harder one works to lose weight through vigorous exercise the more difficult it becomes to control the resulting increase in appetite. Age actually imposes compound forces against an individuals' ability to sustain normal body mass. Apart from the fact that the body's metabolic rate declines with age, physical strength and stamina are also significantly diminished. Moreover, the physical abilities of an obese individual may be significantly less than that of an individual of normal weight.

Equally as important as how much one eats on any given day is precisely when and how frequently this is done. Even if the total number of calories consumed is not significantly reduced, the way in which they are consumed can make a significant impact on how the calories are metabolized. It is certainly better to eat before than after any heavy activity which makes it clear that eating just before going to sleep is not necessarily a good idea. It is also important to understand that when the body is in digestion mode, it burns calories to perform this complex task. In order to do this, a number of physiological tasks are performed to prepare the body. After the food is consumed, the metabolic activities related to digestion continue for several hours until all the nutrients are successfully processed. So, if a long period of time prevails between meals, the entire process must be restarted again. It's sort of like booting up a computer. The computer screen doesn't just pop up when you switch on the computer. It often takes several minutes for all the required software to load before it is ready to be used. It also takes time for a computer to shut down because it must close all open application, save the user settings, install updates and so on. The point to all of this is that eating small meals more frequently keeps the digestive engine from completely shutting down.

Diet and exercise may be considered rather simple and innocuous solutions to the problem of obesity; but, this approach to the problem is easier spoken than done. In addition to shear will power, one must have a plan. This plan must somehow reflect a deviation from the lifestyle that led to the obese state. More often than not, those seeking to lose weight will do so by various means that are not only inefficient and temporary but often very dangerous to their health. Fasting to lose weight can cause serious health problems, including malnutrition, dehydration and possible cardiovascular problems. In similar fashion, vigorous exercise, especially by those individuals who are accustomed to living rather sedentary life styles, can be very dangerous, leading, in some cases to severe cardiac stress and heart attack.

A. The Calorie Counters

Although there are certainly many creative, unscientific ways to lose weight, the most effective way is to precisely regulate the number of calories that are consumed each day. To do this effectively, one must know at least three important things: (1) the number of calories necessary to maintain the target or desired body mass index or BMI; (2) your current weight or BMI; and, (3) the number of calories actually consumed each day. The difference between one's actual BMI and target or desired BMI, when converted to calories, would give the number of calories that must be immediately eliminated from one's daily diet. But doing so does not necessarily mean that the BMI will suddenly drop to the desired level. Remember that the body must burn all of the excess fat in addition to the calories that are consumed even at the lower rate. So, obviously, it will take some time initially to achieve the desired BMI.

It is very important not to shock the body by attempting to achieve one's desired BMI through fasting. In fact, it is much harder to fast than to simply reduce one's daily caloric intake. Instead, a gradual reduction over several months would give the body an opportunity to accept its changing state. Fasting is quite like going "cold turkey", so to speak, if one desires to quit smoking. Indeed, it takes time and concentration to change old habits. With this in mind, let's suppose, for example, that you are accustomed to eating 3,500 calories each day. Now, in order to maintain the desired body mass, you discover that this would require no more than 2,500 calories per day. Rather than to immediately reduce caloric intake by 1,000 calories each day, take your time and diminish your intake slowly, perhaps by 20 calories less each day until you reach the target rate of consumption.

1. The Rule of Ten's

Having offered exciting new suggestions for losing weight through dieting, it may be helpful for the reader to understand a few important rules. It may also be helpful, at this juncture, for the reader to review the computational procedures introduced in **Chapter 1** for the BMI and body fat percentages. Since the concept of calories may be difficult for many to understand it is often more practical to refer to calories in terms of their equivalent in weight. Most of us know what a pound is and how to use it in modern calculations. But, pounds are generally used in the U.S. and perhaps Canada while most of the rest of the world uses kilograms. For the purposes of this discussion we will use pounds; however, for those who prefer it, one kilogram is equal to 2.2 pounds or, conversely, one pound is equal to about .4545 kilogram or one kilogram divided by 2.2.

As a general rule, one pound is equal to about 3,500 calories. So, in order to loss one pound, one must burn away 3,500 calories. Another way of expressing this is by use of what I call the *Rule of Ten's*. Applying this rule, one must burn 10 fewer calories per day to lose about one pound per year or 100 fewer calories per day to lose 10 pounds per year. Conversely, an individual who consumes 100 more calories each day than what the body needs to maintain a normal BMI will gain an additional 10 pounds each year. Applying this rule to a practical example, a person weighing 180 pounds who wants to lose 20 pounds in one year, must consume 200 fewer calories each day. Otherwise, this individual must burn 200 more calories each day through activity or exercise without consuming any additional calories.

The Rule of Ten's is presented to suggest that losing weight by a reduction in caloric intake should be gradual and methodical. But this also depends entirely upon how much weight one really wants to lose over time. For example, a person wanting to lose 20 pounds in three months, based on the Rule of Ten's, would need to consume 800 fewer calories each day, a task that may require considerably more effort, including some vigorous exercise. Nevertheless, losing weight by the Rule of Ten's is not that particularly difficult when you evaluate this in terms of total caloric intake. For example, a person accustomed to consuming 3,000 calories each day who then consumes 2,800 calories to lose 20 pounds in one year has only cut about 14% out of his/her daily food consumption. Moreover, 200 calories per day can be measured very likely in the reduction of just one small portion of food or drink. It can even be measured in terms of the specific type of food that is consumed. For example, instead of consuming 500 calories worth of bacon and eggs for breakfast, one can substitute this for 300 calories of milk and cereal.

2.   The Harris-Benedict Procedure

The Rule of Ten's suggests approximately how many fewer calories it takes to lose weight over a certain period of time. But, in order to derive a specific weight goal, it is also necessary to compute the number of calories required each day to achieve a normal weight at various heights. For example, a normal body mass index for a height of 72 inches is 22. From the computational procedures learned in **Chapter 1**, this equates to a weight of about 162 pounds using a derivative of the Quetelet BMI as follows:

$$Weight = BMI \; x \; \frac{h^2}{703}$$

And;

$$22 \; x \; \frac{72^2}{703} = 22 \; x \; \frac{5184}{703} = 162 \; pounds \; approximately$$

Now that we know how to determine our target weight, it would be helpful to know also precisely how many calories are required to maintain this weight. This will depend upon a number of assumptions. First is that we must know how many calories are burned at rest. You may recall from **Chapter 2** that the body burns calories just to sustain its physiological such as breathing, heartbeat, kidney, brain, liver functions and so on through a process known as basal metabolism. The rate at which calories are burned for basal metabolism is referred to as the Basal Metabolism Rate or BMR. Recall also that this represents about 65% of the body's energy needs. Then we need to know approximately how many calories are burned at various levels of activity and recall that the body also burns calories in the digestive process.

A very useful means of computing minimum daily calorie requirements is by the Harris-Benedict Procedure which was introduced in **Chapter 2**. This method is based on a normal body mass, but can used as a benchmark or frame of reference for those wanting to lose weight. The Harris-Benedict Procedure requires two very simple steps for computing the daily calorie intake requirements for any individual of normal body mass or BMI. The first step requires computation of the BMR (Basic Metabolism Rate). This is accomplished using the following equations for male and female which are offered again as a reference:

For men …

$$BMR = 66 + (6.23 \; x \; W) + (12.7 \; x \; h) - (6.76 \; x \; Y)$$

For women …

$$BMR = 655 + (4.35 \, x \, W) + (4.7 \, x \, h) - (4.7 \, x \, Y)$$

In these equations, W = weight in pounds, h = height in inches and Y = years of age. For example, a 40 year old female who is 65 inches tall and weighs 125 pounds would require a minimum of about 1,316 calories each day for basal metabolism.

The Harris-Benedict Procedure also requires computation of the number of calories burned for various activities. Although there are detailed specific tables of value for various types of activities, the formulas in Table XIII below can be used to approximate calorie requirements for most such activities, based upon a more generalized approach.

Table XIII: Daily Calories Required by Activity Level	
Activity Level	**Total Daily Allowance in Calories**
Little or no exercise (Passive-Sedentary)	BMR x 1.2
Light exercise (1 to 3 days/week, 30 minutes/day)	BMR x 1.375
Moderate exercise (3 to 5 days/week, 30 minutes/day	BMR x 1.55
Heavy exercise (6 to 7 days/week, 1 hour/day)	BMR x 1.725
Very heavy exercise (twice each day, 1 hour each session)	BMR x 1.9

Given the example of the 40 year-old above, if she engages in a moderate weekly exercise regimen, her total daily caloric requirement would be equal to her BMR of 1,316 calories times 1.55 or about 2,040 calories per day. Remember also that we have to add about 11% for thermic metabolism, the number of calories required for digestion, in this case, raising the total to about 2,224 calories.

Suppose now that the 40 year old female in our example actually weighs 140 pounds and that she wants to lose the 15 pounds necessary to achieve a desired weight of 125 pounds. At 140 pounds, her BMR, based on the Harris-Benedict Procedure, would be about 1,382. Assuming that she exercises moderately, adding again the 11% for thermic metabolism, then she is likely consuming about 2,377 calories each day to maintain her present weight of 140 pounds.

The difference between her intake at 140 pounds and the amount required at 125 pounds is a scant 113 calories per day. Despite this, she still wants to lose 15 pounds for a total of about 52,500 calories or equivalent of about 144 calories each day. If she consumes no more than what would be required at a weight of 125 pounds then she would lose about a pound every month.

Putting this all together, we now have two of the three ingredients for a proper weight loss program based on diet. We know how to compute calories for both our desired weight and our actual weight and also the number of calories it takes to burn off a single pound. We also know that we can lose weight either by burning more calories, by consuming fewer calories or both. To summarize, in order to lose one pound, we must somehow burn or reduce our food intake by 3,500 calories. The amount of weight we must lose is the difference between our actual and the desired weight using the following equation: BMR x Activity Level x 1.11. The next step is to determine the actual number of calories there are in the foods we consume.

3. Mapping Calorie Consumption

Among the most cumbersome activities engaged by those desiring to lose weight is to precisely count the number of calories contained in the foods consumed each day. It's difficult enough to do this by measuring calories based on food labels, but to search through mountains of data in a table of calories can be painstaking at best. For those who are content with browsing though tables, **Appendix II**: **Table of Calories by Nutritional Content** is provided, accordingly. Whether using a table or simply measuring content from labels, it is considerably more effective to devise a strict plan of approach that includes predetermined menus from which the caloric content need only be computed once. This menu of selective meals can easily consist of perhaps 20 difference variations or dishes which can be randomly shuffled every week. If we know, for example, all of the ingredients in each of the 20 or so predetermined meals, it is easy to create a personal table of total calories for each such meal.

An important point to consider when regulating one's diet based on randomly selected and prepared meals is that the caloric content of such meals may vary. In fact, the number of calories consumed on any given day may also vary; but, this is acceptable as long as the average daily caloric intake does not exceed the amount that would compromise the desired weight goal. This is especially critical for those dieting under circumstances during which their caloric intake may be compromised during a vacation or business meeting. Indeed, it is much easier to control the content, distribution and timing of meals at home than when on vacation or on business trips eating at restaurants. With this in mind, it is often helpful to include a contingency for an interrupted diet in the overall meal plan. First of all, the meal plan should not necessarily be based on calories consumed per day, but rather upon calories consumed over an extended period such as a month or quarter year. Furthermore, it is important to add a contingency value to the total calories one desires to eliminate from the diet. For example, if we want to lose 5 pounds in three months, this equates to an average of about 194 calories per day. To be safe, it may be necessary to add another 10 or 15 calories to this average in order to account for those days on which it may not be possible to adhere strictly to the chosen diet.

The number of calories contained in food items is now included on the labels of most foods purchased at a typical grocery store. These labels also contain important nutritional information that can help consumers prepare well-balanced meals much more readily. The calorie content of foods is usually given in a suggested serving size. In most cases, this serving size is much smaller than one would generally consume; however, this is done often to make the product appear to have fewer calories. A sample food label is given as **Figure 8** at right. This sample is for macaroni and cheese but is similar to all other labels in terms of its distribution of content. The label is divided among six sections as follows:

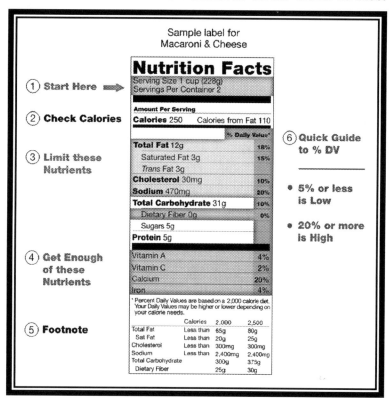

Figure 8: Standard Food Label

(1) the serving size and number servings contained in the package
(2) Provides the total calories per serving, including the number of calories from fat
(3) These are the nutrients that may pose health risks
(4) These are the nutrients of special health value
(5) Footnote indicated
(6) Standard on all labels and provides the recommended daily allowance (RDA) for the nutrients indicated at 2,000 and 2,500 calories

The content food, including total calories, published in labels is not always the total amount that is actually consumed at the dinner table. In the example, a carton of macaroni and cheese may not be enough for the typical consumer. Some may want to add more salt and perhaps some extra cheddar cheese, butter or margarine and/or milk, any or all of which will raise the calorie count. So, it is important when preparing meals to consider all the entrees and the content of each.

B. The Right "Stuff" 'ing

Eating the right foods is equally as important as the total caloric intake necessary to achieve a certain weight goal. It would certainly not be practical to consume 2,000 calories of just ice cream or chocolate cake each day, even if the total consumption is sufficient to actually lose weight. While it's true that one can actually lose weight eating junk food and dessert, the nutritional value of these commodities may not be sufficient to sustain good health. In **Figure 8** at the bottom of the label is an important table that appears on most nutritional labels (note that proteins are missing from the figure, but this is covered below). These are the recommended daily allowances or RDA for the primary nutrients required by the body. The reader may recall from **Chapter 2** that, even though the consumption of fat contributes to obesity, the body needs it for cell protection and lubrication. Carbohydrates are needed for energy, so without them, it would likely be difficult to exercise. The body also needs protein for cell repair and construction. Then, of course there are the dietary fibers, minerals and vitamins.

The specific distribution of food content, in terms of the appropriate proportions of fats, proteins and carbohydrates, should be roughly the same whether dieting as a vegetarian or otherwise. Although vegetarians generally do not eat meats, especially red meats, they must still obtain the recommended daily allowances for dietary fat. Dietary fat, including cholesterol and saturated fats, can come from many other sources besides meat. For example, milk and certain type of nuts contain a significant amount of dietary fat. A popular source of food for many vegetarians is soy bean and the many derivatives thereof, but the calories contained in soy beans actually consist of 40% fat, mostly unsaturated fat. Another 35% of the calories contained in soy beans come from protein and most of the rest from carbohydrates.

1. Recommended Daily Allowances (RDA)

Barring specifically all of the many ingredients of various foods, it is easier to focus simply upon the percentage of nutrients that should be consumed each day. Since these are measured usually in grams and milligrams, it would be easier to convert these allowances to calories and percentage to the total daily allowance for the important nutrients such as fat, protein and carbohydrates. We already know that there are about 3,500 calories in a pound. We should also know a few other things. First is that that one pound is equal to 453.6 grams. Second is that one gram of fat has nine calories while proteins or carbohydrates each have four calories per gram. Finally, more than 99% of the calories consumed each day come from fat, protein and carbohydrates so we needn't worry too much about the rest. It should also be understood that many of the other nutrients, including the vitamins and minerals required each day are generally contained in the three primary nutrients.

Table XIV: Recommended Daily Allowance at 2,000 Calories

Nutrient	Quantity in Grams	Calories	Percentage
Total Fat (includes 20 grams of saturated fat and .3 grams of cholesterol)	65	585	29.25%
Sodium	2.4	0	0
Potassium	3.5	0	0
Carbohydrates	.3	1,200	60%
Fiber	25	15	.75%
Protein	50	200	10%
Total	**146.2**	**2,000**	**100%**

Now that we know the percentage of nutrients recommended each day, counting calories by the RDA standards is just a matter of applying the math. For example, if we want to have a baked potato, by itself even cooked, it only has about 130 calories, but most of it carbohydrates. In fact a typical 150-gram potato contains 26 grams of carbohydrates and 4 grams of protein. So, now where are the other 120 grams? Indeed, it is very important to understand, when reading food labels that the total weight value of food really has very little to do with calories because a lot of it is water. The 122 grams or about 80% of the weight of a typical potato is actually just water which has no calories. When we add up the calories by what's contained in a potato, there are (26 x 4) = 104 calories worth of carbohydrates and (4 x 4) = 16 calories from protein for a total of 120 calories.

Not too many will consume a potato by itself and certainly not raw. Most will add something else for taste. For example, it is very common to add butter to a baked potato. Unfortunately, one ounce of butter has a whopping 203 calories, most of this, about 99%, from fat. Adding this to the total, a baked potato with just one ounce of butter will be 253 calories worth of food. If sour cream is added to the total, one ounce of sour cream contains about 60 calories of which 50 are from fat. Thus, a baked potato with an ounce of butter and another ounce of sour cream will contain 313 calories of which about 81% consists of fat calories. Since the RDA for fat is only about 30%, this enriched potato will have consumed almost half the daily allowance of fat given a 2,000 calorie diet.

It was interesting to discover that a typical baked potato is about 80% water. In fact, just about everything we eat consists mostly of water. The volume of a typical whole fryer chicken, for example, consists of about 60% water. With this in mind, a pound of chicken will contain about 9.6 ounces of water. About 55% of a quantity of ground beef will be water. The leaner the beef, or the less fat it contains, the higher will be its percentage of water. So, why is this all so important? Well, water is what gives foods its general bulk (not to be confused with fiber) and is also what helps to overcome hunger impulses. A significant component of the hunger impulse is that feeling of fullness one gets when the stomach expands after a meal. Water is also a factor in accurately evaluating weight loss and gain. A diet too much in salt content will tend to cause the body to retain fluids for a longer period thus contributing possibly to an overstatement of one's actual weight. On the other hand, the consumption of alcohol, which acts like a diuretic, can cause temporary dehydration and understate one's actual weight.

Because water has no calories, it is important when reading food labels, to understand that calories refer only to the solid contents of what is being consumed. For example, an eight-ounce container of concentrated chicken noodle soup is only about 33% solid food from which calories are derived. Consequently, the actual physical weight of food does not translate to human body weight, except only temporarily until the body has dispelled the fluids through the skin and kidneys. It takes considerably longer for the fluids contained in foods to be dispelled than it does a glass of water, soda or beer. Bearing this in mind, the best time to check body weight or stand on a scale is early in the morning before breakfast or after waking from a long sleep.

2. The Glycemic Index

The reader may recall from **Chapter 2** how carbohydrates are metabolized to produce glucose for energy. Glucose can be obtained not only from carbohydrates but also directly from eating foods high in sugar content. For example, the glucose derived from eating a potato will take almost eight times longer to process than what is obtained from a candy bar. A candy bar is loaded with carbohydrates in the form of sugar; but, sugar is a simple carbohydrate. It is a simple carbohydrate because it requires very little if any digestion to be converted into glucose. The reason for this is that sugar, like glucose, is a saccharide. Glucose is actually a monosaccharide and sugar (table sugar), a disaccharide. So, table sugar is actually made up of two monosaccharides which are easily and quickly converted to the more basic monosaccharide. Potatoes and similar foods high in carbohydrates, including breads and rice, are classified as complex carbohydrates because they must be reduced by several digestive hormones and in several stages to be converted finally into glucose.

Even though certain foods may be considered as complex carbohydrates, they too will vary in the rate by which they are converted to glucose. This is an important distinction because the slower this rate of conversion, the lower will be the body's demand for insulin. The reader may recall from **Chapter 2**, that insulin is released by the pancreas to regulate the production of glucose. Recall also that too much glucose in the blood, known as blood sugar, is a symptom of Type 2 Diabetes. The rate by which carbohydrates are converted through digestion to glucose is referred to as *The Glycemic Index* (GI). The GI is actually a means of classifying foods, in particular, carbohydrates, by the rate at which they are converted to glucose. The higher this index, the faster the rate of conversion and also, the greater will be the risk of raising the body's blood sugar levels. As a general rule, the standard Glycemic Index is a value falling on a range between 0 and 100; however, some Glycemic charts have GI values as high as 140. The important thing to remember is that Glycemic charts are typically presented with foods that are high, medium or low in their Glycemic value. A GI value of 55 or less is considered low. A GI value falling between 55 and 70 is medium or average, but any GI value greater than 70 is considered high.

The Glycemic Index of foods can be influenced significantly by the way in which they are prepared, what they contain and how they are consumed. For example, foods high in fiber will usually have a lower GI. Foods high in fat and protein content will also slow the digestion process and thus lower the GI. For example, even though potatoes are complex carbohydrates they have a high GI by themselves, but when served with butter and/or sour cream, can actually be consumed with a lower GI. It is also interesting to note that foods high in acid content such as lemon juice and vinegar will tend to lower the GI. This is an important distinction considering that the acidity of foods decreases with age. For this reason, ripened fruits will usually have a higher GI than un-ripened or freshly harvested fruits. **Table VX** below gives a sample of common foods and their Glycemic Index.

Although the Glycemic Index is itself an important value for determining the rate by which foods containing carbohydrate are converted to glucose, it does not account for the actual serving size. For this reason, it is necessary to convert the GI to an equivalent that accounts for this, a value known as the *Glycemic Load*. In order to find the Glycemic Load of a particular food, divide the GI by 100 and multiply the result by the number of grams of carbohydrates (less the grams of fiber) as shown on the food label. The Glycemic Load index falls on a range from zero to 20. Any value less than 10 would be considered low, but any value greater than 20 would be considered high. For example, a ¼-cup serving of white rice contains about 35 grams of carbohydrates. Given its GI value as shown in Table XV, the Glycemic Load would be (70 ÷ 100) x 35 = 24.5 and quite high. The same quantity of brown rice has 33 grams of carbohydrates after you subtract out the fiber content, but its GI is only 55; thus, its Glycemic Load index would only be (55 ÷ 100) x 33 = 18.15, and still on the high side of normal.

Table VX: Abridged Glycemic Index Table							
Breads, Grains & Cereals		**Legumes & Starchy Vegetables**		**Fruits and Snacks**		**Dairy, Sugars and Beverages**	
Item	**GI**	**Item**	**GI**	**Item**	**GI**	**Item**	**GI**
Oatmeal	58	Raw Carrot	31	Raisins	64	Whole Milk	21
Doughnut	76	Baked Potato	78	Banana	51	Skim Milk	32
Whole Wheat Bread	73	Mashed Potato	73	Orange	48	Ice Cream	62
Wheat Bread, White	69	Sweet Potato	48	Apple	40	Table Sugar	65
Bagel	72	Baked Beans	40	Grapes	43	Soft Drinks	63
Brown Rice	55	Split Peas	32	Potato Chips	57	Orange Juice	46
Rice, White	70	Kidney Beans	23	Oatmeal Cookies	54	Apple Juice	41
Spaghetti	41	Soy Beans	15	Chocolate	44	Beer	0
Corn Flakes	77	Butter Beans	36	Corn Chips	42	Ice Tea	0
Shredded Wheat	67	Lentils	28	Peanuts	13	Coffee, cream, sugar	21

3. Timing is Everything

The digestive process is indeed a very complex mechanism and one that certainly takes its time to process what we eat. Now imagine putting solid food in a blender in order to render it into a liquid or creamy substance. If all of the food is thrown into the blender at once, it will clog up or simply just blend what's closest to the blades. In this instance, it would be necessary either to remove some of the content or to push it down with a wooden spoon closer to the blades. This is certainly not a practical way of using a blender. The best way, in fact, is to gradually add food to the blender as it is churning it away. This process may take a bit longer, but will likely do so with fewer complications. This analogy raises the point why one should chew food thoroughly and slowly before actually swallowing it because it is a mechanical means of improving the efficiency of digestion.

Very much like the blender, if we eat a very large meal and do so very quickly it will take the body much longer do digest it, and it will do so with much less efficiency. What happens is that the body will overproduce hormones, especially insulin, to meet the demand until those hormones are dispelled. Meanwhile much of the food is either passed as waste or, because of the increased blood-insulin levels, it is stored as fat. Eating such a large meal late or shortly before bedtime can make matters even worse considering that, during sleep, the body's metabolism is significantly slowed. At the same time, the body's thermic metabolism is working overtime to digest the late meal. This action contributes to restless sleep, sleep apnea, snoring and even insomnia.

Given the preceding discussion, it is only logical to conclude that eating several smaller meals throughout the day rather than one large meal allows our digestive process to operate more efficiently. In fact, all such meals should be consumed sufficiently early with the last meal of the day consumed at least three to four hours before going to sleep. Many dieticians recommend eating a large breakfast, moderate lunch and a small dinner, each about four hours apart. Unfortunately, by sheer habit, most Americans do quite the opposite. This habit was borne, not so much from tradition, but out of necessity, especially in modern times. Indeed, breakfast is usually touch-and-go because Americans are rushed to get to work. Lunch is small and quickly consumed because of the short rest period that is usually allowed to prevail for this activity. What's left is dinner, the meal at which most of us make up for what was missed during breakfast and lunch. Then there is, of course, the "midnight snack" or dessert. These are consumed habitually just before going to bed.

C. When and How to Exercise

Having learned a bit about how to regulate our eating habits, it often helps to construct a plan of physical exercise, especially for those who are not too thrilled about dieting. While exercise often overcomes binge or too much eating, it can also significantly reinforce the process of losing weight and then help to preclude gaining it back again. Exercise should actually become a habit, something that is done on a regular basis, for the same duration of time and usually at around the same time of day. But exercise, like controlling one's diet, comes with many surprising caveats. The most alarming among these is the fact that, in some cases, one can actually gain more weight by exercising. With this in mind, one wonders why we should even bother to exercise at all. Well, aside for the health benefits associated with exercise, it will help us to indeed lose and control weight if we understand and manage the complications of this activity.

The three major complications associated with exercise are (1) physical risk of injury and/or cardiac stress; (2) increase in muscle mass and (3) increase in appetite. The intended benefit of exercise, when done so to lose weight; however, is to increase the body's activity metabolism in order to burn more calories. But, this can only happen if everything else is either held constant or reduced. In other words, exercise would be meaningless if more calories are consumed accordingly. Even if the exercise is not coupled with planned diets, the intake of calories one is accustomed to should not increase at all. When diet and exercise are adhered to strictly then weight loss would have to occur by default. The reason for this is that fewer calories are being consumed while at the same time the increase in activity metabolism from exercise actually burns more than the usual number of calories. Suppose, for example, that a usually sedentary individual consumes an average 2,800 calories per day. Let's also assume that this person decides to reduce daily consumption to 2,500 calories per day and exercise enough to burn an average 300 calories per day. If this individual sustains this regimen without interruption, it could result in a weight loss of about five pounds every month or 1.2 pounds per week.

The major risk associated with exercise applies usually to those who are not accustomed to it. A sedentary individual who suddenly decides to jog three miles each day is risking serious cardiac stress because the body has not been trained to handle the sudden surge in activity metabolism. If this individual is obese, the risk of cardiac stress is even higher. You see, an increase in activity metabolism will also affect basal metabolism through increased respiration and cardiac output. It is very important for the reader to understand that everything, including exercise must come in moderation and by this means can actually convert health risks to health benefits. This means that any plan to lose weight must be associated with a gradual, not sudden, increase in activity. Instead of immediately jogging three miles each day, it is better to walk a mile every other day for a week then perhaps increase this to every day or increase the walk distance another mile each week. After several weeks of this moderate exercise regimen, then start by jogging one mile every other day and increase this regimen to a daily routine or increase the distance another half mile each week until a daily jogging regimen of three miles has been achieved.

Exercise will always increase muscle mass, a process called the anabolic effect, because more muscle is required to provide the body the strength it needs for this activity. Increased muscle mass comes with two, often unintended side effects. First of all, as more muscle mass is accumulated through exercise, this may actually result in an increase in one's weight. The myth about muscle is that it is believed to actually weigh more than fat, but it really doesn't. Fat is just not as concentrated or as dense as muscle. To be fair, however, when measured as an equivalent unit, a cup of fat weighs less than a cup of muscle. When an individual exercises to burn off fat, this is replaced or offset with more muscle mass. In other words it is quite possible through exercise to lose a pound of fat but gain a pound of muscle in the process. Another point to ponder is that, because fat is not as dense as muscle, a pound of fat will take up considerably more body area than a pound of muscle. For example, a pound of fat occupies almost twice the amount of space than does a pound muscle which is why fat people appear so large. The other unintended consequence of exercise may apply more to women than to men. Exercise tends to build muscle girth and bulk. Women who want to appear feminine or dainty would certainly not be happy with how increased muscle mass can make them appear more masculine instead.

The most elusive side effect of physical exercise is that it requires more energy to which the body responds with an increase in appetite. For this reason, it is often helpful to exercise before instead of after a meal without actually increasing the caloric content of the meal consumed. Unfortunately, the number of calories burned during exercise is often more than offset by the voracious appetite that can result from this activity. As a general rule, one should exercise either in the morning before breakfast or early in the evening before dinner without actually increasing the amount of calories consumed. It is certainly not a good practice to exercise after a meal even though it may appear to be a logical thing to do. First of all, exercise will significantly slow the digestive process because the body's activity metabolism will interrupt its thermic metabolism. The reason for this is that exercise increases the body's demand for energy from all sources. It's sort of like shutting down all non-essential systems in favor of the essential systems during a power outage. Furthermore, after the exercise is completed, even if this activity is engaged after a meal, there will still be a resulting increase in appetite.

A final point regarding exercise is that this activity really doesn't burn as much as one might expect. For example, as vigorous and as potentially dangerous as jogging may be, a 180-pound individual jogging three miles in 20 minutes will only burn about 375 calories. The actual intensity of the activity held constant, the more we weigh the more calories we will burn. With this in mind, a 300-pound man will burn more than twice the calories as a 150-pound man provided that both perform at the same rate. Unfortunately, heavier individuals will likely be considerably more sluggish than those who are of normal weight simply by the sheer force of their own weight. This is also yet another reason why exercising after rather than before a meal is not recommended. For the convenience of the reader, a comprehensive table of activity calories is provided as **Appendix III**.

D. Chapter Summary

Diet and exercise are the two most obvious and commonly employed methods for managing obesity. The purpose of diet and exercise is to reduce the body's consumption of calories sufficiently to burn off excess body weight. In order to do this, a specific plan of approach must be undertaken which includes a determination of the daily required calorie consumption to sustain a specific weight.

In order to lose one pound, the body must burn 3,500 calories, preferably over an extended period of time. By the Rule of Ten's, it takes 100 fewer calories each day to lose 10 pounds in one year. The number of calories that must be burned each day to achieve the desired weight goal can be computed using the Harris-Benedict Method.   By this method, a recommended weight-loss plan would be to reduce daily caloric intake by the difference between the calories required to maintain one's current wait and one's desired weight.

The number of calories consumed each day can be obtained from most food labels which also include recommended daily allowances or RDA for fat, protein, carbohydrates and other nutrients. Carbohydrates and protein each contain 4 calories per gram and fat, 9 calories per gram. There are 453.6 grams in one pound. More than half or about 60% of the daily caloric intake should consist of carbohydrates; another 29.25% should consist of fat; 10% of protein and the rest of fiber.

Carbohydrate intake should consider the rate by which it is actually converted to glucose by a value known as the Glycemic Index or GI. The GI rates carbohydrates on a range from 0 to 100 on most scales. A GI value of less than 55 is consider low and one greater than 70 is considered high. A more important value which takes into account the actual amount of carbohydrates consumed is known as the Glycemic Load. This value is computed by dividing the GI by 100 and multiplying the result by the carbohydrates contained in the foods we eat less their fiber content. The Glycemic Load should not exceed 20.

Exercise is beneficial as reinforcement for any plan to lose weight through dieting; however, exercise can impose certain health risks, actually result in weight gain from muscle mass and increase appetite. Taken in moderation and about the same time each day, exercise should be performed regularly before and not after meals.

Key Points:

1. One pound of body weight is the equivalent of one calorie
2. By the Rule of Ten's, in order to lose about 10 pounds in a year, one must reduce food consumption by 100 calories per day
3. By the Harris-Benedict method the daily required calorie intake is computed as follows: BMI x Activity Level x 1.11
4. The daily RDA of caloric intake includes 60% carbohydrates, 29.25% fat, 10% protein and .75% fiber
5. The rate by which carbohydrates are converted to glucose is determined by the Glycemic Index (GI)
6. The higher the GI the greater will be the likelihood of raising blood-sugar levels
7. The Glycemic Load is equal to the GI divided by 100 times the amount of carbohydrates (less fiber) contained in foods
8. It is more beneficial to consume several smaller meals each day than one large meal late in the day
9. The last meal of the day should be consumed at least three to four hours before going to bed
10. Exercise can burn calories as long as the daily caloric intake is not increased as a result.
11. Exercise should be undertaken in moderation to avoid cardiac stress
12. Exercise can increase appetite and muscle mass

Chapter 9--*Non-Medical, Alternative Approaches to Managing Obesity*

The basic problem that plagues most of us when confronted with the challenge of losing weight is that we either do not have the time or we don't have the motivation. Otherwise, the physical and sociological constraints upon our daily lives simply make it impossible or impractical. Dieting and exercise takes persistence, regular and often precision planning which are almost invariably interrupted by the mere trials of daily life. For those who travel a lot and those whose jobs require the entertainment of customers, dieting is virtually impossible. Moreover, there are many individuals who can diet but simply cannot exercise because they may be handicapped. Then there are those who can only diet and exercise on weekends, when on vacation or perhaps only after they retire. Whatever the constraints, it is clear that not everyone possesses the means to diet and exercise "by the book" so to speak.

Those who can't diet and exercise or those who simply won't may often seek short cuts or other creative means of achieving their weight goals. Some will restrict their diets exclusively to protein, carbohydrates or both, completely eliminating fat, but take multi-vitamins, herbs, minerals and supplements to help overcome the nutritional deficiencies that may result. There are also those who rely on specially prepared medications to help control or to diminish their urge to eat. This type of treatment is referred to as homeopathic medicine in which very small, but decreasing doses of certain substances are administered over a long period of time to help control cravings and to also improve digestion and hormone balance. Then there are also those who seek help through more controversial methods such as psychotherapy, hypnosis and acupuncture.

The most common reason that diet and exercise are not sustained is a lapse in motivation. Indeed, when confronted with the problem of obesity one is initially motivated, either by external stimuli or by self-induced will. But it doesn't take long to discover that perseverance is easier celebrated than actually sustained. In the military, soldiers must be motivated by strict rules of conduct, order and dress, as well as by the will of their leaders. They are pushed well beyond the physical limits of most individuals and definitely well beyond even what they as individuals perceive they can accomplish. Self-motivation is difficult, even for Type A, highly aggressive individuals, especially if they do not know the limits of their own capabilities. For this reason, a multibillion dollar industry emerged from which numerous diet and exercise programs have emerged on television, DVD, website and books. There are literally dozens of well-known celebrities who have developed entire careers just in helping motivate people to diet and exercise. But, as they say, "You can lead a horse to water ..." so it often even takes personal trainers and motivators to get the job done.

A. Homeopathic and Other Alternative Treatments

Many believe that the chemicals used by pharmaceutical companies to manufacture drugs do more harm than good. Even though there are numerous published contraindications and known chemical interactions associated with various drugs, scientists still do not really know precisely how some drugs react to the natural chemicals and hormones in our bodies. Since the chemicals in drugs are invariably metabolized in the liver, long-term use of these substances can cause serious and irreparable damage to this organ. These and the many other risks associated with manufactured chemicals have led many individuals to seek alternative approaches for treating their maladies.

Although many alternative medical approaches to obesity will include the prescription of certain specialized drugs or chemicals, most involve the judicious use of herbs, nutritional supplements and behavioral therapies. If drugs and chemicals are indeed used, they are done so in small, water soluble dosages

1. Homeopathy

One very useful method of treating obesity is by a prescribed regimen of specially prepared supplements or chemicals taken over time, but in successively reduced dosages through a process called *serial dilution*. This type of approach to managing obesity is known as *Homeopathic Medicine*. A typical homeopathic treatment protocol begins with the administration of small doses of plant, animal or synthetic substances, most of which help to control cravings and accelerate digestion. Over time, the dosage of these supplements is reduced, often without the patient's knowledge, until the prescription is essentially nothing more than a placebo (inert substance). The process for creating homeopathic substances is controversial at best. The reason for this is that it usually involves the use of chemicals, organic components or certain elements which produce symptoms similar to those of the condition being treated. It's sort of like fighting fire with fire or, in this case, fat with fat, quite consistent with the adage that a cure can be derived from consuming "The hair of the dog that bit you". But many believe it to be a form of witchcraft by which treatments are prepared from bazaar sources such as the waste or byproducts of a disease process.

Despite its controversial evolution, homeopathic treatments appear to have worked in many cases; albeit, many doctors dispute the validity of these successes. Unlike the "hard" drugs, most of which are used to specifically treat a condition by killing invading organisms, regulating hormones and enzymes or treating disease symptoms, homeopathic medicine is intended to augment or stimulate the body's own defense mechanism or immune system. It does so in the treatment of obesity by somehow controlling the various hormones that regulate appetite, fat metabolism and insulin production. But many doctors argue that, even in maximum dosages, the treatments are nothing more than placebo and only work if such treatments somehow psychologically induce a cure. Homeopaths argue that this is precisely what their drugs are intended to do—to induce a sort of autoimmune reaction. Whether or not this is a chemical or psychologically induced reaction really doesn't matter as long as the intended outcome is achieved. A list of some of the more common homeopathic substances used in the treatment of obesity is given in **Table XVI**.

Table XVI: Common Homeopathic Substances and their Use in Treating Obesity	
Substance	Claim
Antimonium Crudum	Used to treat irritability, especially when dieting
Argentum Nitricum	Reduces cravings for sweets
Calcerea Carbonica	Reduces appetite and helps calm nerves
Coffee Cruda	Helps to reduce anxiety and depression
Capsicum	Treats face flush and heartburn during digestion
Graphites	Helps to control weight gain in menopausal women
Ignatia	Helps to reduce anxiety, depression, nervousness
Lycopodium	Controls cravings for sweets

2. Herbs and Supplements

If you think about it, the key to losing weight is to curb appetite, increase the body's rate of metabolism (activity metabolism) or to do both. So, if it is not possible to achieve this through controlled diet and exercise, there are other means, although not nearly as effective. Indeed, certain herbs and supplements, most of which are manufactured from substances contained in plants, roots and tree bark, can somehow actually help to control appetite and to accelerate metabolism. But, herbs and supplements are not necessarily a cure-all. Taken by themselves they may help to achieve one's weight loss objective; but, in order to optimize their effectiveness, at least some regimen of diet and exercise would be necessary.

Among the most important supplements that can help control appetite is fiber. Recall that fiber is very little more than a medium that carries food through the body's alimentary canal (digestive system). Fiber has no calories, but is actually non-digestible bulk that helps to overcome the feeling of emptiness that comes with hunger. It does so in two ways. First is that it adds bulk or quantity to whatever foods that contains it. Bulk in food expands the stomach making us feel full. Secondly and more importantly is that fiber actually helps to lower insulin levels which also helps to make us feel fuller. Fiber also promotes efficient digestion and helps to eliminate bulk waste. In fact, fiber is often referred to as roughage in that it helps to eliminate or prevent the onset of constipation. Fiber can also help to control diarrhea in that it provides a medium for the absorption of fluids. **Table XVII** below gives a list of the most common herbs and supplements used in the management of obesity

Table XVII: Common Herbs and Supplement Used in Treating Obesity	
SUPPLEMENTS	
Conjugated Linoleic Acid (CLA)	Helps to reduce body fat and enhances lean body mass
5-Hydroxytryptophan (5-HTP)	Helps to inhibit appetite or hunger cravings by boosting serotonin levels in the central nervous system
Zinc	Works a lot like CLA to sustain lean body mass and reduce fat
Chitosan	Made from shellfish as a fiber supplement
Pyruvate	Increases production of lactic acid which in turn increases metabolism
Hydroxycitric Acid (HCA)	Helps to prevent carbohydrates from being stored as fat
Glucomannan	Helps to reduce blood sugar levels and increases metabolism of stored fat
HERBS	
Psylium	A highly soluble fiber that helps reduce hunger cravings
Green Tea	Increases metabolism and thus helps to burn stored fat
Gogul	Helps to reduce weight by diminishing appetite and increasing metabolism
Cayenne	Suppresses appetite
Hoodia	Controversial substance, not really considered an herb, but arguably useful for suppressing appetite

3. Other Obesity Treatment Methods

When all else fails, there are still other non-medical alternatives to losing weight. Some of these are more radical than others.

- **Acupuncture**: a Chinese method by which needles are inserted into various locations of the body to stimulate the production of serotonin levels thus helping to suppress appetite
- **Hypnosis**: a highly controversial method in which subliminal suggestion is used to induce motivation or simply to suppress appetite. Hypnosis makes no hormonal changes but can change mental perceptions to the point that certain brain hormones are altered to suppress appetite
- **Cognitive Behavioral Therapy**: this method involves interaction with a trainer, therapist or support group as a means of encouraging healthy behavior that may result in weight loss
- **Home Remedies**: these include a number of surprising ways to lose weight.
  - Honey taken with lime juice and lukewarm water when hungry
  - Regular intake of carrot juice helps to suppress appetite
  - Eating a tomato after breakfast every morning suppresses appetite
  - Cooked cabbage in lieu of a regular meal for increased metabolism
  - Mint taken with every meal will help suppress appetite
  - Grown curry leaves every morning helps suppress appetite
  - Luke warm, boiled ginger and lemon suppresses appetite
- **Dynamic Tension**: a type of exercise done without too much effort such as squeezing the hands and arms together, pushing one hand against the side of your head or moving your knees together in a sitting position while pulling them apart with your hands.
- **Meditation**: Because stress and anxiety can contribute to obesity, meditation is often an effective way of dealing with these emotional issues. Meditation involves deep concentration and relaxation for at least 30 minutes at a time.
- **Massage Therapy**: Massage therapy is intended to stimulate blood circulation. This helps the lymphatic system to eliminate toxic waste and also increases the production of gastric hormones. Massage therapy is also effective at managing stress.
- **Sweat Therapy**: When the body sweats, it actually eliminates toxins and waste. Many of these toxins are known as free radicals or oxidants which tend to interfered with normal digestion and hormone function. Obesity also causes oxidant stress which can lead to cardiovascular disease.

B. Brown Fat

Unlike the bulky, irregular white fat that permeates the bodies of overweight individuals, there is another kind of fat that is found primarily in new born infants and hibernating mammals. This fat is known as brown fat, so called because of its high concentration of iron. What is so unique about brown fat is that it really isn't stored in the body for future digestion as energy. In fact, brown fat actually burns through white fat and is used to regulate body temperature. This remarkable discovery has become a focus of broad research in the way that brown fat can be used as a tool to combat obesity. Even though brown fat is diminished as we grow into adulthood, some still remains in our bodies throughout life. It was discovered that the amount of brown fat that our body retains appears to be much higher in cold than in warm temperatures. This follows from the fact that brown fat regulates temperature and may account for its increased presence in hibernating mammals. It is also interesting to note that there is considerably more brown fat per unit of body mass in individuals of normal weight than those who are obese. Moreover, women are more likely to store brown fat than men and, in fact, store almost twice as much.

The challenge that remains in regard to brown fat is just how its presence can be accelerated to help reduce weight from white fat. Scientists now know that brown fat seems to be much more prevalent in individuals when they are cold than when they are warm and comfortable. This interesting discovery led to a practice by some individuals to regularly dive into and swim in icy water, sometimes for as long as an hour in each session. In fact, the practice of taking a cold shower every day is believed to actually result in weight loss over time according to a study conducted by researchers at the University of Maastricht in the Netherlands. Based on the results of this study, taking a cold shower once each day for a year can result in weight loss of as much as nine pounds; however, this outcome appeared to be more prevalent in women than in men.

Apart from exposure to cold as a means of activating brown fat, research really hasn't disclosed a so called "magic pill" to activate it at will. Instead, scientists do know that there are certain activities which can actually suppress the production of brown fat. Cessation of such activities can at least help to sustain the levels of brown fat that exist naturally in the body. For example, eating the right quantities of food slowly as suggested in the previous chapter can help to sustain brown fat while either under-eating or over-eating can suppress brown fat activity. Eating foods high in sugar content or dining on low-fat diets can also suppress brown fat activity. Even stress, anxiety and depression can suppress brown fat activity. Surprisingly, too much exercise can also suppress brown fat activity.

C. Fad Diets and the Machine Age

Having asserted this several times previously, it is important, again, to understand that the only way to lose weight is to either reduce calorie intake or to increase metabolism. It really doesn't matter how this is done as long as it is understood that one must simply burn more calories than are consumed until the weight goal is achieve. The fundamental problem that most individuals have with the prospect of losing and controlling weight is just how to do this easily, quickly and effectively. Diet and exercise require determination, discipline and perseverance. Homeopathic and alternative health methodologies are controversial and piecemeal. Then there are, of course, the diet fads, dozens of them!

Diet fads tend to be more a source of financial success for those who promote them than of any benefit to the lay consumer. In fact, it's a multi-billion dollar industry. But, all that these fads really do is to operate on human emotion by their often extraordinary claims of instant success. Many such fads come with weight loss guarantees; but, these guarantees usually only warrant initial and not sustained weight loss. Since weight loss requires the body to burn more calories than consumed, the way most fad diets work is to eliminate or reduce fat-producing nutrients or to add fiber and useless, calorie-free bulk to the diet. In either case, you basically eat as much as you're used to eating, but consume fewer calories.

In addition to the billions of dollars spent by consumers on diet fads, there is also virtually every type of exercise equipment imaginable to help them along. Like the diet fads, the promotion of exercise equipment preys upon the consumers need for immediate and successful weight loss. Such promotions make the same extraordinary claims and guarantees as do those for the diet fads. The problem with exercise equipment is that it represents a major financial investment in something which, if not used, does nothing but collect dust. Remember that "…you can lead a horse to water."

1. The Diet Revolution

Diet fads are simply just big business and most do not really achieve the desired results. The diet fad industry, in fact, had earned an average $40-billion each year since 2005; but, obesity continues to prevail despite the industry's financial success. The industry is successful because it offers fast and methodical results, but at a hefty price. The way in which most of these fads work is to get you join a club for a monthly fee. The fee includes three specially prepared meals each day and lot's of promotional material and offers from other companies. Some companies go so far as to offer internet or telephone support groups and others encourage the formation of local support groups. These groups conduct periodic meetings or so called "pep rallies" to help motivate customers to stick to their diet plans.

What many who buy into these diet fads do not realize is that the companies who promote them are doing very little more than operating upon the many principles discussed in this book. For example, a typical diet fad is the quintessential "low-carb diet". With this diet, one is basically offered a supply of specially prepared meals low in carbohydrates, but at price usually higher than it would cost to prepare the same meal at home. Fewer carbohydrates may result in weight loss because most of the excess stored fat in our bodies comes from undigested carbohydrates. Because fewer carbohydrates are consumed, in order for the body to obtain its energy, it must draw it from stored fats; hence, weight loss may result. What really happens, however, is that the fewer carbohydrates or offset by more fat and protein. Too much fat causes obesity and too much protein causes other problems such as protein poisoning.

There are also other types of fad diets, equally as controversial as the common, low carbohydrate diet. For example, the so called "low-fat diet" is intended to completely eliminate fatty foods especially those containing saturated fats, transfatty acids and hydrogenated fats. While one may think that eliminating fat can result in weight loss, it really doesn't. If you recall the discussion on brown fat above, remember that too little fat in one's diet can actually suppress the production of brown fat. Brown fat burns through white fat. Remember also that the body needs at least 29.5 grams of fat daily according to RDA guidelines. White fat is needed by the body for cell insulation and protection, so the total elimination of this nutrient can suppress the body's immune system.

Another popular fad is the "protein diet". With this diet, only foods high in protein content are consumed. This diet is really a combination of the low-fat and low-carb diets in that very little, if any, fat or carbohydrates are consumed. The problem with protein diets is that, while such diets can achieve weight loss goals, their unintended consequence is protein poisoning. After being on a protein diet for long periods, protein poisoning can result. Protein poisoning can cause fatigue, diarrhea, headache, low blood pressure and heart rate and vague hunger. The vague hunger symptom can only be relieved by consuming more fat and/or carbohydrates. In fact, many who are on the protein diet will have almost insatiable cravings for fatty and starchy foods and thus are in constant temptation to compromise their diet regimen.

Bulk diets are also popular. A bulk diet is one that is high in water or fiber content. The idea behind these diets is that they simply help overcome hunger symptoms. With these diets one can basically eat the customary amount of food but with fewer calories per meal. Remember that neither fiber nor water contains any calories. The problem with these diets is that they often taste bland and unappetizing. Consequently, those who manufacture the meals associated with such diets will add higher doses of sodium, monosodium glutamate and other chemicals to improve their taste.

2. Rise of the Machines

It's not enough to pay hefty fees for consumer diet fads. Remember that a diet without exercise is perhaps like bread without butter. Even though walking, jogging and biking are excellent ways to exercise, many individuals do not live in areas where this is possible. Those who live in urban or cold environments usually must confine their exercise to some type of indoor activity. In this case, a nearby gymnasium, a mall or the stairs in a high-rise apartment complex may offer suitable alternatives, especially for vascular exercises. The solutions in these instances is to … well … walk or run in place, do push-ups and sit-ups and maybe some jumping jacks. Otherwise, a TV or DVD exercise program might be useful. Indeed, the need for effective and convenient exercise accommodations has actually given birth to several other lucrative industries. Among these are the myriad health clubs, private gymnasiums and exercise clinics. Then, of course, there is the fitness equipment. Like the diet fad industry, fitness equipment is a lucrative business. In fact, the fitness industry in 2010 amassed a whopping $2 billion, almost triple its earnings in 1980.

The use of specialized equipment is often an effective way to exercise and there are certainly a myriad of choices available from simple compression devices to complex, all-in-one machines. Some are even compact and portable enough to be carried on business trips or vacation. The really good machines, especially those that are multi-functional are usually very expensive and take up a lot of space. The multifunction machines are also very complex and take time to change from one mode to another. Many exercise machines, unfortunately operate only on one muscle group. To overcome this problem, many individuals will then buy more machines to handle the other muscle groups. Many serious individuals will purchase weight lifting machines, treadmills and stationary bicycles and other equipment, all of which could occupy an entire 120 square feet of area or larger.

Not only is fitness equipment sold in the primary market, but also in the after or secondary market. Many health clubs and private gymnasiums will upgrade their equipment periodically, selling their old machines to companies that clean and refurbish them for resale. There are also companies which buy and sell used equipment from individuals who eventually lose patience or interest in the equipment. In both cases, the equipment is bought at a significantly reduced price, often less than 15% of its original value. Then it is resold often at a price not too far removed from its price when it was new. Some fitness equipment, especially treadmills and similar such electronically controlled devices often require periodic maintenance and repair at additional cost.

The alternative to buying and storing expensive fitness equipment conjured yet another lucrative industry—health and fitness clubs. For a monthly fee, fitness clubs offer access to all sorts of fitness equipment plus the attention of professional trainers. Many fitness clubs also offer group exercise programs such Pilates, aerobic dancing and Qi gong. The group exercise programs offer a disciplined approach to exercise much like it is done in the military. Pilates is a highly specialized exercise form developed in the early 20th century in Germany by Joseph Pilates. Pilates are exercises that place the body in focused, strained or balanced positions, a technique which requires deep concentration and controlled breathing. The objective of Pilates is to improve cardio vascular function and develop deep torso muscles. Aerobic dancing is very popular because it is sort of recreational in nature. Because it involves an aggressive, dance-type regimen, aerobic dancing burns calories quite as effectively as jogging or biking. Aerobic exercise in general not only burns calories but also helps to improve and sustain cardiovascular health. Qi gong is a type of group exercise which originated from ancient Chinese martial arts practices such as Kung Fu and Tai Chi Chuan. Qi gong is believed to help blood circulation and thus increase metabolism.

D. Chapter Summary

There are many alternative, non-medical approaches to managing obesity. Unlike diet and exercise, however, the purpose of these methods is to either accelerate metabolism or to inhibit appetite. Among these is homeopathic medicine, a method by which small doses of a substance known to cause certain symptoms in healthy individuals are administered in serial reduced quantities. This method as well as certain herbs and dietary supplements can be taken to help control appetite and increase body metabolism. Aside from ingesting dietary aids to controlling obesity, some individuals may seek more esoteric approaches to controlling their weight, such as hypnosis, group therapy, acupuncture, sweat therapy, meditation and even certain homemade remedies such as warm green tea with honey, cooked cabbage and carrot juice. But, even radical application of these treatments regimens should still be accompanied by regular dieting and exercise to be effective.

Scientists have recently discovered a type of metabolic fat known as brown fat which actually eats through the white fat that accumulates to make us obese. Occurring primarily in newborn infants and hibernating mammals, brown fat appears to be activated when individuals are exposed to cold weather. This discovery was confirmed by a study by researchers at the University of Maastricht in the Netherlands, who determined that a cold shower taken daily for one year actually resulted in an average weight loss of about nine pounds.

Another way to manage obesity is through the strict and regimented diet plans of the myriad diet fads that comprise a multi-billion dollar industry. Diet fads make use of prepared meals, most of which contain fewer calories because they are served with high concentrations of fiber, water and other non-caloric bulk. The general principal behind such diets is to eliminate hunger stimuli without the expense of excess calories. Another multi-billion dollar industry consists of companies that manufacture and sell a variety of exercise equipment to individuals, public and private gymnasiums, health clubs and fitness centers. Most such equipment focuses specifically upon certain muscle groups and some of the more complex fitness machines can be very expensive, cumbersome to use and difficult to store. The alternative to buying bulky exercise equipment is to join a health club. The advantage to health clubs is that most have a variety of fitness machines and devices as well as certified and specialized trainers. Fitness clubs also provide group exercise programs such as Pilates, aerobic dancing and Qi gong.

Key Points:

1. Alternative approaches to losing weight include those methods intended to either control appetite or increase body metabolism
2. Brown fat is a naturally occurring adipose tissue in the body that is known to actually metabolize or burn through common white fat
3. Brown fat can be activated by exposure to cold such as swimming in cold water or taking a cold shower
4. Homeopathy, herbs and supplements are believed to help control or reduce appetite or increase body metabolism
5. Hypnosis, meditation, acupuncture and similar such methods are designed to help eliminate stress and anxiety which are both underlying precursors of obesity
6. Diet fads make use of prepared meals containing large concentrations of bulk such as water and fiber to help control appetite at a smaller expense in calories
7. Personal exercise and fitness equipment provides a controlled and focused means of developing certain muscle groups but can be expensive, cumbersome and take up lots of space
8. Fitness and health clubs provide access to a variety of fitness machines, personal trainers and group exercise programs such as aerobic dancing, Pilates and Qi gong.

Chapter 10--*Medical & Surgical Management of Obesity*

When all else fails and one has exhausted every conceivable approach to managing obesity, including diet, exercise and the myriad non-medical approaches to suppressing appetite and increasing the body's rate of metabolism, it may be time for a trip to the doctor's office. Indeed, there are many cases of obesity which simply cannot be effectively managed except through interventional medicine. The medical and surgical management of obesity are certainly in the last frontier of alternatives to the problem; but, they come with many risks and unintended side effects. Medical intervention can also be very expensive and many insurance plans do not cover the cost even though the interventional outcomes can preclude the onset of the more serious, obesity-related medical problems such as Type 2 Diabetes and cardiovascular disease.

The medical and surgical management of obesity can be as simple as drug therapy or as complex as surgical reduction of the stomach. Many doctors who are confronted with the management of obese patients will try to avoid surgical intervention initially. Sometimes they may reassure their patients that diet and exercise, as well as the alternative medical approaches, should be tried first. If these have been tried to no avail, doctors will begin by prescribing certain medications to help increase metabolism and suppress appetite. If this doesn't work, they may try hormone therapy. They may even recommend cosmetic surgery such as tummy tucks and liposuction, in all cases, hoping to avoid the most extreme intervention—invasive surgery.

A. Dietary Pharmacology

Referring again to the central objective of obesity management, in order to lose weight, the body must burn more calories than are actually consumed each day. The underlying principle that governs this objective encompasses one or both of only two fundamental approaches—(1) suppression or regulation of appetite and (2) the acceleration of body metabolism. Appetite is regulated traditionally by the strict adherence to a prescribed quantity, composition and frequency of a specified diet. The traditional approach to increasing body metabolism is simply to exercise more. Otherwise, there are numerous non-medical approaches to weight loss. But, when none of these seem to help manage the problem, a little help from the local pharmacist may be in order.

The use of drugs to manage obesity is a field of specialization known as *dietary pharmacology*, a clinical approach the treatment of this condition that makes use of chemical agents or so called "anti-obesity" drugs to suppress or restrict appetite, regulate the digestive process and/or increase the body's rate of metabolism. Dietary pharmacology also includes the administration of drugs which act as fat substitutes or inhibitors. These chemicals are intended to significantly reduce the fat content of foods without diminishing the "creamy" consistency or taste associated with fats. Although dietary pharmacology is considered an effective alternative to the traditional approaches to weight loss, because it involves the ingestion of processed and/or synthesized chemicals it may impose unintended side effects.

1. Appetite Suppressants

Drugs used to suppress appetite are categorized generally as *anorectic agents*. These agents are used typically in conjunction with certain behavioral therapy to help inhibit or suppress hunger stimuli. Anorectic agents are divided into two distinct groups of drugs that were actually specifically engineered as antidepressants. The first of these are called *noradrenergic agents* which help to suppress appetite by inhibiting the release of the neurotransmitters dopamine and norepinephrine, hormones which act to make us feel hungry. The second group consists of drugs called *serotonergic agents* which inhibit the release of serotonin. Recall that serotonin is the hormone that helps to regulate the actual amount of food eaten by increasing *satiety*, the feeling of fullness. Appetite suppressants, in general, do not necessarily affect the physiological character of digestive metabolism. Instead, they act on the brain to affect certain neuro-stimuli that alter human perception, emotion and senses. The perceptions that affect how much an individual eats include (1) hunger or appetite and (2) satiety or the point at which an individual is full or no longer hungry.

The principal anti-obesity drug used to suppress appetite is phentermine, a drug approved by the U.S. Food and Drug Administration (FDA) which acts on the brain to increase the release of norepinephrine. Although norepinephrine controls the fight-or-flight mechanism of human behavior it is also released to suppress appetite or signal the brain to convey perceptions of satisfaction after a meal. When the levels of norepinephrine begin to decline, this causes an individual to develop feelings of hunger. Consequently, a drug-induced increase in the level of norepinephrine before a meal has been known to help suppress appetite in most individuals to whom phentermine has been prescribed. Phentermine also acts to release adrenaline which helps to accelerate the break-down of stored fat. The reported side effects of phentermine include headache, tachycardia or elevated heart rate and short-term, elevated blood pressure.

Another popular anti-obesity drug is an FDA-approved product called *subutramine* or Meridia which is a serotonergic agent that works on the brain receptors to make an individual feel full or less hungry after consuming even small amounts of food. The feeling of fullness after a meal is actually a neurological defense mechanism known as satiety. If the brain was not made aware that the stomach is full, hunger pangs would continue, thus causing someone conceivable to keep eating, quite to the point at which this activity can become fatal. Most patients who are prescribed subutramin drug are reputed as having lost 5% to 10% of their body mass in less than one year. Although the drug is somewhat effective by itself, ancillary weight loss activities such as diet and exercise are generally recommended. Long term use of subutramine can cause hypertension, elevated heart rate, headache, constipation, dryness of the mouth and insomnia. Many physicians believe that the action of this drug in increasing heart rate may actually result in weight loss from an increase in metabolism; however, an elevated heart rate at rest can lead to cardiac arrest.

2. Thermogenic Agents

When the body burns calories, this mechanism actually causes a rise in body temperature. This is among the reasons the metabolic process used to describe digestion is known as thermic metabolism. Drugs used to artificially accelerate body heat to increase thermic metabolism are known as thermogenic agents. These agents increase heart rate and blood pressure to accelerate *thermogenesis*. Thermogenesis is the process by which organisms produce heat. Among the more effective protocols used to increase thermogenesis is a cocktail combining caffeine with a drug called ephedrine. Ephedrine by itself works much like appetite suppressants to release norepinephrine, but when administered with caffeine can significantly augment thermogenesis thus increasing thermic metabolism and the number calories burned during digestion. The side effects of this cocktail are quite similar to those one experiences after drinking too much coffee. These may include tremor, dizziness and insomnia.

3. Digestive Inhibitors

Another clinical approach to managing obesity through drug therapy is to actually interrupt or somehow inhibit the metabolism of dietary fat. This is done by somehow bypassing the absorption of triglycerides so that they are passed into the large intestine before actually being absorbed into the blood stream. The principal drug used to inhibit digestion is orlistat or xenical. Although orlistat is quite affective at inhibiting the digestion of body fat, it does so at a cost. Long-term use of orlistat can result in fatty stools and frequent diarrhea. This in turn can result in a decrease in the body's electrolyte balance, increase in heart rate and elevated blood pressure.

4. Fat Substitutes

The fundamental problem with obesity is that it results from the accumulation of too much adipose tissue or fat. Even though the body needs a certain amount of fat for heat insulation and cell protection, there is certainly plenty of this in overweight individuals. Consequently, the elimination of fat entirely from the diets of obese individuals will invariably induce the body to metabolize stores and quite to the point that weight loss will occur. But, who wants to eat foods without fat? Fat is what gives many foods their creamy and moist texture. Fat also makes it a lot easier to swallow foods, albeit, less likely to efficiently chew such foods before they are swallowed.

In order to eliminate fat without actually eliminating the taste and consistency of fats, it is possible to combine certain foods with an additive or so called "fat substitute". A popular such additive is a product called olestra. Made from sucrose polyester, olestra acts just like fat but bears a molecular structure that is far too large to be absorbed into the blood stream. In fact, olestra works almost precisely like fiber in that it has no calories and is simply passed out into the stool. Olestra is considered very effective at inducing weight loss because its use requires the body to obtain its essential triglyceride nutrients from stored fats. The problem with olestra is that its use makes it almost impossible for the body to absorb the fat-soluble vitamins A, D, E and K. Consequently, patients prescribed with olestra must also take vitamin supplements to overcome this deficiency.

B. Hormone Therapy

Having read **Chapter 2** of this book, it should be clear that the entire digestive process is really very little more than a long chemical reaction. This reaction consists of a blend of various nutrients in the foods we eat with hormones released during the digestive process. These hormones are released in order to break the food down to a state that is easily absorbed into the blood stream. Because we understand how hormones work to aid in the digestion of food, we have also found ways to somehow regulate their behavior through various external means. Among these is the use of drugs to help suppress appetites as was discussed in the previous section of this chapter. Appetite suppressants work primarily on the brain to stimulate the release or inhibition of certain digestive hormones. With hormone therapy, on the other hand, synthetically manufactured hormones are taken orally or by injection in order to increase their presence in the body. The hormones used primarily for treating obesity include T3 and T4 thyroid hormones and surprisingly, both progesterone and testosterone.

The reader may recall from **Chapter 3** how the thyroid gland can misbehave by either an overproduction or underproduction of the T3 and T4 hormones which regulate metabolism. An increase in T3 and T4 will actually induce a condition known as hyperthyroidism which coincidentally can result in weight loss from an increase in body metabolism or the rate by which the body burns calories. Synthetic T3 and/or T4 are often prescribed for the treatment of hypothyroidism, a condition resulting from an underproduction of these hormones. Consequently, in an obese individual who does not suffer from hypothyroidism, the administration of these hormones can actually have therapeutic benefits. T3 and T4 can be prescribed by a physician or obtained over-the-counter in the form of desiccated or freeze dried thyroid. Most prescriptions for thyroid hormones consist only of the T3 component because many patients do not respond well to the T4 component. Given in combination with T3, the T4 hormone can cause ankle swelling, heart palpitations, insomnia and, in some cases, increase in appetite.

Recall that testosterone is a hormone found in both males and females. Aside from its function in male sexuality, testosterone also plays a major role in the metabolism of fat in and around the abdomen. As a result of the aging process, the levels of testosterone, as well as those of progesterone, can begin to deplete. This can result in a dominance of a third group of sex hormones known collectively as estrogens. Estrogens exist in both males and females, but are more important in regulating sex drive in females. Estrogen dominance is particularly evident among menopausal and post-menopausal women in whom it can cause weight gain and fatigue. In males, estrogen dominance can result in an increase in the production of breast mass and abdominal adipose accumulation or the so called "beer belly". Synthetic testosterone administered regularly to both male and females can significantly reduce the effects of estrogen dominance.

Progesterone is a hormone found primarily in females and is released especially during pregnancy, birth and regularly to control the menstrual cycle. Progesterone levels usually begin to deplete significantly from aging during the menopausal and post-menopausal stages of adult life. We already know that decreased progesterone levels can result in estrogen dominance which can cause obesity. But, one important function of progesterone is to regulate the thyroid gland. As progesterone levels decline, this can cause the depletion also of the levels of T3 and T4 resulting in hypothyroidism and reduced metabolism. The administration of synthetic thyroid hormones, as well as synthetic progesterone, is quite effective at restoring hormone balance.

C. Cosmetic Solutions to Obesity

For many who are obese, rather than spending perhaps months and even years to lose weight through substantial restrictions in their lifestyles, they may seek help through cosmetic means. Cosmetic solutions to the management of obesity are sought by individuals for various reasons such as peer pressure, career growth suppression, marital strife, vanity or an inability to lose weight by any other means. For these individuals, weight loss through radical cosmetic intervention may be the answer. Cosmetic solutions to obesity can be quick and effective, but are largely controversial because of the potential harm they can cause, not only in physical appearance but also in one's health. Many of the more effective cosmetic interventions are also quite expensive and most are not covered by health insurance plans.

Obesity-related cosmetic intervention is intended not only to surgically remove or dissolve excess body fat but also to help deal with the ugly skin folds, stretch marks and wrinkles that result from having lost a significant amount of weight. No matter how it is accomplished, rapid weight loss can leave the skin sagging for an intolerably long time. Although human skin is quite resilient, it loses much of its elasticity, firmness and smooth texture as the body ages. Just as the skin of a woman stretches during pregnancy, so too will it stretch to provide space for excess fat. As skin stretches, it gets tighter and harder as what may happen when you inflate a balloon or rubber raft. After an immediate surgical reduction in weight, the skin is left dangling and will take many months to contract into the smaller body mass that results.

There are several alternative approaches to the cosmetic removal of excess fat. Among these is the ever-popular, very effective but controversial lipoplasty or liposuction whose namesake derives literally from the fact that fat is removed through a tube very much like a vacuum cleaner. There are several different approaches to liposuction, each used in accordance the condition and tolerance of the patient. Another approach is to dissolve fat or reduce the appearance of ugly cellulite scars through a procedure called lipodissolve or mesotherapy. Unlike the more aggressive liposuction, fat dissolution is really a non-surgical approach which makes use of certain chemical solutions beneath the skin to remove fat.

1. Liposuction (Lipoplasty)

The most effective means of removing excess fat through cosmetic treatment approaches is liposuction, or more scientifically, lipoplasty. Liposuction is a procedure by which a surgeon makes a small incision and then inserts a hollow straw-like tube called a *cannula* just under the patient's skin. This tube is attached to type of vacuum or suction device known as an *aspirator*. Moving the hollow tube back and forth under the skin, a process called *subcutaneous agitation*, the surgeon breaks up the fat so that it is easily passed or sucked up into the tube. Before undergoing this procedure the patient is rendered comfortable with a sedative and local anesthetic; however, some patients may be administered general anesthesia depending upon their tolerance and also upon the extent of the procedure.

Liposuction is not usually done all at once because it can be a dangerous and traumatic experience. Instead, small amounts of fat, usually no more than 5 to 8 pounds at a time are removed over the course of several procedures during several weeks or months. Radical liposuction has been reported in which as much 50 pounds was removed in one session. If too much fat is removed in one session, this can be potentially life-threatening in that it represents an untoward shock to the system. The procedure must also be done methodically in usually one area at a time to avoid the appearance of lump irregularities under the skin.

There are several alternative liposuction approaches each of which differs only in the way fat is processed or broken down before it is passed into the cannula. In most cases, the physician will inject small amounts of solution mixed with a local anesthetic. This numbs the area while at the same time creating a space between the muscle and fat tissue, thus helping to minimize post-surgical bruising. The key to performing a successful liposuction procedure is to break the fat down into simple, almost fluid-like material that is easily drawn into the cannula. Otherwise, the cannula, as well as the aspirator, can become clogged. One method of doing this is by the use of ultrasound which actually emulsifies the fat or renders it down into an oily fluid. The advantage of ultrasound-assisted liposuction as this procedure is called is that it is much faster than the traditional approach and requires less agitation by the surgeon. The disadvantage is that excessive ultrasonic stimulation can cause damage to surrounding tissue. It can also increase the incidence of *seroma* formation. A seroma is pocket of fluid just under the skin which must be managed through post-surgical drainage using a needle and syringe.

Subcutaneous agitation of the cannula is a potentially dangerous technique in that a careless surgeon can easily puncture organs or, in the case of abdominal liposuction, inadvertently cut through the peritoneum. A breach of the abdominal peritoneum can result in serious complications, including infection. For this reason, other specialized surgeons may be present during a liposuction procedure. An effective innovation that avoids potential injury from manual agitation is twin-cannula liposuction or TCL. In this case, there are two cannulas, one within the other. The outer cannula acts like a shroud which is inserted under the skin. The inner cannula is actually a reciprocating tube which mechanically agitates the fat and then draws it into the aspirator. TCL is considered among the safest approaches to liposuction; however, the rapid reciprocating action of the inner cannula can cause friction burns.

There are many side effects associated with liposuction, most of which subside within several weeks. The most obvious of these are post-surgical bruising and swelling. Depending upon the extent and nature of the procedure, there may also be some scarring. Pain is also very common and is usually managed with buffered pain medication. In some cases, liposuction may cause temporary disfigurement, especially with liposuction of the face and neck. Of course, skin folds, stretch and tiger marks and other skin irregularities will be very apparent and may in some cases require plastic surgery to tighten, especially in older patients. In many cases, patients may require psychological counseling to help them cope with their initial appearance following a liposuction procedure.

2. Mesotherapy (Lipodissolve)

An alternative to the radical liposuction procedure is to eliminate fat by simply dissolving it and allowing the body to remove the resulting waste naturally. This is done by means of a process called mesotherapy, a non-surgical treatment in which fat-reducing solutions are injected under the skin to dissolve or convert fat so that the body considers it very little more than expendable waste. Mesotherapy is also sometimes known as lipodissolve, although the latter is considered one of several different approaches to mesotherapy. With mesotherapy, various solutions of pharmaceutical, homeopathic, plant extracts, vitamins and supplements are injected frequently over an extended period. The injected solution induces a mechanism known as *lipolysis*, the destruction of adipose cells called *adiposytes*.

Although mesotherapy is known to achieve results in most reported cases, it is highly controversial in that much of the content of the solutions used in the procedure are not FDA-approved. Consequently, the procedure is largely experimental. Mesotherapy is very commonly used in Europe, but is viewed with much consternation by the medical community in the United States. In fact, the American Society of Plastic Surgeons rails on the procedure and has actually issued formal statements denying its clinical efficacy. Nevertheless, many dismiss such statements as the product of medical provincialism.

3. Tummy Tucks (Abdominoplasty) and Other Methods

Most individuals who are overweight will begin developing the characteristic or so called "beer" gut around the lower abdomen. In fact, the lower abdomen is where most adipose tissue usually begins to collect. In obese and morbidly obese individuals, of course, adipose tissue will collect not only in the lower abdomen but also under the upper arms, around the hip, buttocks and thighs and in the face and neck area. But, the belly is usually where most of the fat likes to hang out or, put more descriptively, hang over. Belly fat is also an obvious characteristic of overweight individuals. But, belly fat is not just fat that accumulates under the skin. It can also wrap around the intestines, liver and other abdominal organs.

There are a number of ways to manage belly fat, but the quickest and most expedient way is to have it surgically removed. This is done in one of several approaches classified collectively as abdominoplasty or, very simply, the "Tummy Tuck". The most radical approach to the tummy tuck is to draw an incision laterally across (not down) the belly, reach in and remove as much fat as possible and then carefully suture the incision to minimize scarring. This procedure works very much like caesarean section (C-section) for complicated childbirth except that the incision is only skin deep. For women concerned about post-surgical scarring, the tummy tuck procedure can be accomplished via a bikini cut. On the other hand, a mini tummy tuck is a way of removing abdominal fat through a small, single incision to the lower abdomen.

Tummy tucks result almost invariably in scarring because the excess skin must be removed and then tightened before being sutured back together. Otherwise, a large flap of skin will remain until it eventually shrinks or recedes, a process that could take months. In many cases, tummy tucks may require the repositioning of the belly button which, for women, may not be a desirable outcome. Nevertheless, because of the cosmetic nature of tummy tucks, they are usually performed by highly trained plastic and reconstructive surgeons.

While tummy tucks are intended to remove fat, there are also several cosmetic procedures necessary to help manage the results of immediate weight loss. Liposuction, tummy tucks and even radical weight loss through diet and exercise will certainly eliminate fat quickly, but the skin remains, droopy, wrinkled and saggy. In fact, many patients develop feelings of anxiety and depression just from their unsightly appearance following excessive weight loss. Many believe they look much older and unfortunately may often gain all the weight back again. It is important to understand that what happens to the skin after significant weight loss is much like what happens after giving birth. The skin will eventually shrink back and restore its healthy look, but this will take many months. The alternative, of course, is plastic surgery.

Plastic surgery helps to eliminate the unsightly folds, wrinkles and sagging skin that results from losing weight rapidly. With plastic surgery, an incision is made in various areas of the body where fat had accumulated, excess skin is cut away and the skin that remains is pulled tight and sutured closed. Plastic surgery is especially effective under the chin, the buttocks, upper arms and under the breasts. The purpose of plastic surgery is not necessarily to remove fat but to restore the skin back to its tight and healthy appearance quickly following rapid weight loss from various surgical procedures.

D. Surgical Management of Obesity

The last and most radical frontier of approaches to the management of obesity is surgical intervention. Unlike cosmetic surgery which applies primarily to the subcutaneous (just under the skin) regions of the anatomy, surgical management involves the invasive (pertaining to the internal organs of the body) modification of the stomach, duodenum and small intestines. Surgical management of obesity is recommended usually for those who are dangerously or morbidly obese and those who could otherwise die if their obese condition is not surgically resolved. There are a number of approaches employed in the surgical management of obesity all of which are collectively referred to as *bariatric surgery*.

Bariatric surgery consists of several alternative approaches to digestive intervention that can be classified into two distinct groups. First among these are the *malabsorptive bariatric procedures* which are intended to help restrict the absorption of nutrients into the blood stream. As a result, patients who undergo these procedures will lose weight since a large portion of what they consume will be passed as waste instead of being absorbed into the blood stream and stored as fat. The second group consists of the *restrictive bariatric procedures*. These involve restricting by clamping or simply reducing the size of the stomach the result of which is intended to help reduce hunger and appetite.

Bariatric surgery is generally very expensive because of the potential co-morbidities and complications that can occur with these procedures; however, because they are essentially considered emergency interventions, most are covered by insurance plans. Nevertheless, most insurance companies will carefully evaluate patients undergoing bariatric surgery to determine whether or not they are seeking such intervention for cosmetic reasons. If so, the procedures are not generally covered. But, for morbidly obese patients, especially those with advanced complications associated with Type 2 diabetes, those with severe and chronic hypertension and those with serious cardiovascular complications associated with obesity, most plans will cover the procedure.

1. Malabsorptive Bariatric Surgery (MBS)

The underlying principal behind malabsorptive bariatric surgery (MBS) is that, by restricting the absorption of nutrients, no matter how much is consumed by the patient, most of it will be passed into the stool as waste instead of being absorbed into the blood stream. Consequently, the body must obtain the nutrient deficiencies from excess fat, thus resulting in spontaneous weight loss. The problem with these methods is that they can lead to serious malnutrition and vitamin deficiency. Consequently, MBS is usually intended for morbidly or dangerously obese patients and is done so only temporarily. These procedures are done as short-stop measures and reversed after the patient has lost enough weight to begin leading a normal, healthy life.

An MBS procedure gaining widespread attention in the medical community is a rather complex gastric by-pass known as the duodenal switch with vertical gastrectomy. With this procedure, a large portion or about 70% of the stomach is first removed creating a much smaller stomach. Removal of the stomach in this way is called a *gastrectomy*. Then the duodenum and jejunum are detached from the stomach, but not from the common bile duct and pancreas. This insures that the transfer of digestive hormones is not interrupted. In order to by-pass the jejunum, about 150 centimeters of the distal (the end) part of the small intestine or ileum are cut away and then attached to the stomach where the duodenum and jejunum were detached; however, the end of the jejunum is attached to the by-pass just before it enters the caecum. The

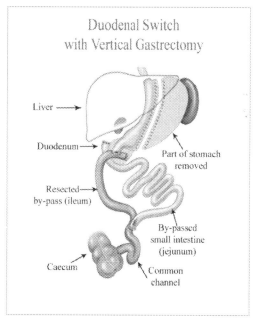

Figure 9: Duodenal Switch Procedure

length of ileum from this junction to the caecum is called the common channel. The purpose for attaching the jejunum thusly is to insure that some digestion and absorption occurs within this channel. The duodenal switch procedure is illustrated in **Figure 9**.

Because a large portion of the small intestine is removed with the duodenal switch procedure, much of the food that is consumed cannot be absorbed into the blood stream and is instead passed on as waste. As a result, significant weight loss occurs rather quickly because the body's need for energy is obtained from fat stores. With this procedure, only about 20% to 25% of the nutrients that are consumed are actually metabolized. For this reason, the diets of duodenal switch patients must be supplemented with compensatory amounts of vitamins, minerals and supplements. Some patients may also need appetite suppressants because the body will tend to overcompensate for nutrient deficiencies by triggering the hunger stimuli.

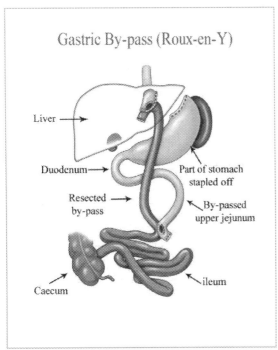

Gastric By-pass (Roux-en-Y)

Liver

Duodenum

Resected by-pass

Part of stomach stapled off

By-passed upper jejunum

Caecum

ileum

Figure 10: Roux-en-Y gastric by-pass

The most popular and commonly performed MBS procedure is the *gastric by-pass*, also known as the Roux-en-Y procedure. In many respects, the gastric by-pass procedure is quite similar to the duodenal switch in that it by-passes the duodenum and a large section of the jejunum. Instead of performing a gastrectomy, however, all but a small portion of the stomach is stapled leaving a small stomach pouch close to where the esophagus enters the stomach. Then the small intestines that were cut away from the duodenum and upper jejunum are attached to the remaining stomach pouch. The cut away duodenum and jejunum are attached to the by-pass at the lower jejunum or upper ileum where digestion resumes. This alternative MBS procedure eliminates most of the stomach, the duodenum and the upper jejunum where a large share of the digestive process occurs. Consequently fewer nutrients are digested sufficiently to be absorbed into the ileum and lower jejunum and are thus passed as waste. **Figure 10** illustrates the Roux-en-Y procedure.

Other more radical malabsorptive approaches to bariatric surgery include the *jejunoileal by-pass* in which almost the entire small intestine is by-passed altogether and the *endoluminal sleeve procedure* by which an impermeable synthetic tube is surgically inserted into the duodenum and upper jejunum to help restrict absorption. The jejunoileal by-pass procedure is no longer performed because it can result in severe malnutrition. The endoluminal sleeve procedure, however, is often preferred over the duodenal switch procedure because it does not require extensive by-pass and resection of digestive organs. On the other hand, the procedure only blocks about 20% or less than a third of what can be accomplished with the duodenal switch procedure.

2. Restrictive Bariatric Surgery (RBS)

The principal objective of restrictive bariatric surgery (RBS) is to diminish the size of the stomach. By so doing, the feeling of fullness is achieved with much smaller quantities of food. RBS procedures are considered much safer than the MBS alternatives in that normal digestion and absorption are not affected. The disadvantage of RBS is that patients having undergone these types of procedures will digest their smaller quantities of food more quickly and thus tend to eat more frequently to compensate. For this reason, many physicians will reinforce the RBS procedure with post-surgical prescriptions of appetite suppressants.

The most commonly prescribed RBS procedure is the vertical gastroplasty, often also called the Mason procedure or just simply "stomach stapling." With this procedure a large portion of the stomach is permanently stapled, thus leaving a small so called "stomach pouch". The same thing can be accomplished using an adjustable gastric band, the use of which precludes having to make an incision into the stomach. The adjustable gastric band procedure as this is called makes use of a flexible band which is wrapped around the upper portion of the stomach and drawn tightly, like the hand squeezing the top of an inflated balloon. This leaves a small stomach pouch between the band and where the esophagus enters the stomach. The way it works is that the food enters this small stomach pouch until the pouch is full. This signals the brain to stimulate that feeling of fullness or sateity. Meanwhile the food is very slowly passed into the larger area of the stomach like sand through the neck of an hour glass and eventually digested. This band is flexible in that its diameter, or the tightness by which it constricts the stomach, can be adjusted by injecting a saline solution into it through an easily accessible subcutaneous port.

Another approach to reducing stomach capacity is to insert an inflatable, intragastric balloon endoscopically. An endoscopic procedure is one in which a tube is passed into the body in one of several different ways, orally down through the esophagus and into the stomach, a procedure known as a gastroscopy, via a small incision through the abdominal cavity, a procedure known as a laparoscopy and many others. This tube has a mini camera or scope (why it's called "-scopy") attached to its end so that the surgeon can observe the course of the procedure via a closed-circuit television monitor. The balloon is inserted in a deflated state then inflated with a saline solution to the desired size. Because the balloon takes up a significant amount of stomach space, only a small capacity remains to contain food. Consequently, the feeling of fullness is achieved much more quickly.

A more radical approach to stomach reduction is a procedure known as the sleeve gastrectomy. Since it's a gastrectomy this means that a portion of the stomach is surgically removed. What remains are two flaps which are sutured together to form a sleeve, thus leaving the stomach much smaller and having the appearance of a banana. The sleeve gastrectomy has the same effect as all of the other stomach–reduction procedures except, unlike the adjustable gastric band procedure, it leaves the stomach permanently reduced in size.

E. Chapter Summary

When all of the traditional and non-medical approaches to weight loss fail, the last frontier available to those who are desperate to solve their problem with this condition is to visit the doctor's office. Although most physicians will attempt to exhaust all non-medical avenues including the recommendation of diet and exercise, they will first attempt to manage the problem through many available anti-obesity drugs. These include appetite suppressants, thermogenic agents to reduce hunger, digestive inhibitors to prevent the absorption of large portions of the food that is consumed and fat substitutes which are low-calorie binders that taste like fat. The physician may also prescribe hormone therapy to manipulate the hormones that regulate appetite, hunger and digestion.

There are also various cosmetic surgical procedures available, most of which are engineered to surgically remove or dissolve fat or to cosmetically restore flabby and loose skin to a healthier appearance. Cosmetic surgery is risky, as well as costly, and most such procedures are not covered by health insurance plans even though they may prevent more serious health problems. Moreover, cosmetic surgery does not really treat the problem. Instead, it only resolves the outcome of whatever underlying circumstance may prevail that caused the obesity problem in the first place.

The absolute last resort to weight loss is one or a combination of several types of an invasive intervention called bariatric surgery. Bariatric surgery may inhibit nutritional absorption through bariatric malabsorptive surgery (BPS) or accelerate the feeling of fullness after a meal by means of the restrictive bariatric surgery (RBS). The BPS procedures involve bypassing the duodenum and portions of the small intestine to prevent digestive absorption of a large percentage of the food that is consumed; however, these procedures can cause malnutrition and vitamin deficiency. The RBS procedures involve a reduction in the size of the stomach so that the feeling of fullness is achieved after consuming only small amounts of food.

Key Points:

1. Dietary pharmacology consists of the administration of drugs to suppress appetite, eliminate or suppress hunger or to intervene in the digestive process
2. Dietary hormone therapy consists of the manipulation of hormones that control appetite, feelings of hunger and digestion
3. Cosmetic intervention is intended to surgically eliminate or to dissolve excess fat and to help restore the skin to its normal state following immediate weight loss
4. Malabsorptive bariatric surgery (MBS) is done to reduce the amount of nutrients absorbed into the blood stream by surgically bi-passing the duodenum and small intestines

5. Restrictive bariatric surgery (RBS) is done to reduce the size of the stomach so that the feeling of fullness is achieved after only a small meal

Epilogue

As of the publication of this book, prevailing research continues to underscore the notion that obesity might not be entirely one's fault. Aside from the fact that obesity may even be contagious or contracted from the proliferation of certain bacteria or genetically predisposed, it is likely also that this condition can be either caused or exacerbated by industrial chemicals. In fact a recent study highlighted in The New American Diet, by Stephen Perrine and Heather Hurlock revealed that many of the foods we eat are processed by the use of what the authors refer to as "obesogenic" substances such as pesticides, plastics and other chemicals. These substances may alter the hormonal balance of the body quite to the point of making us obese.

Two notable "obesogens" are phthalates and bisphenol (BPA) both of which are chemical derivates used in food containers. Phthalates are found in certain cosmetics, PVC pipe and medical tubing and bisphenol can be found in baby bottles. Although the studies are not conclusive, evidence is mounting which points to the industrial complex as a source of chemically-induced obesity. What plagues medical science specifically about the notion of "obesogens" is in clinically understanding and explaining the etiology or mechanism by which such chemicals can trigger the onset of obesity. What scientists do know is that certain chemicals, such as those used in pharmaceuticals can induce changes in the body's delicate metabolic and hormonal balance.

Recent studies conducted by the University of California, San Diego suggest that obese children are more likely to develop antibodies to adenovirus AD36 which causes some strains of the common cold as well as certain types of eye infections. In fact, children with antibodies to AD36 were about 50 pounds heavier on the average than those who did not have the antibody. Researchers believe that AD36 may actually rewire the fat cell structure thus contributing to obesity in children. If scientists can establish a link between obesity and AD36 in terms of a causal relationship, treatment protocols could be developed to effectively combat childhood obesity.

Another recent discovery distinguishes between those who eat to live and those who live to eat. Indeed, some individuals are actually predisposed, according to recent studies, to an insatiable desire to eat, not because they are glutinous or because they lack the will to control themselves, but because of the way in which the chemicals of their brains react to the stimulus of certain foods. These individuals are categorized into a functional pattern of brain stimuli known as the hedonic mechanism of hunger. Those in this category are known as hedonic eaters. At the opposite end of the extreme are those who eat simply to survive. These individuals are grouped into the category of homeostatic eaters. The latter group is considered functionally normal in that the members of this group tend to possess normal chemical reactions to hunger and appetite.

In order to understand the difference between homeostatic and hedonic eaters it is important to distinguish first between hunger and appetite, both related yet remarkably different. Hunger is actually triggered by a natural mechanism in our bodies and occurs more specifically when the levels of glucose in the blood stream decline below normal levels. Hunger is also induced by contractions that occur in the lining of the stomach when it is empty. Theoretically, when the stomach is full and glucose levels rise to normal, the feeling of fullness, or what is referred to as satiety, should induce the cessation of eating.

Unlike hunger, appetite is more a function of how the brain reacts to the stimuli of foods such as their appearance, taste and smell. The brain's reaction to foods can actually be environmentally influenced by a broad range of stimuli, including advertising, social convention or community behavior and even force of habit (conditioned response). Well known Russian physiologist, Iven Petrovish Pavlov was the first to introduce the notion that our brains can be trained to respond habitually to certain stimuli if such stimuli are associated with pleasure or pain. Using dogs in an experiment to test their reactions, Pavlov associated the sound of bells with the food that they ate. After many trials, the dogs became intuitively reactive to food each time the bells were rung. Even when the food was removed from the experiment and even during short intervals between meals, when the bells were rung, the dogs salivated as if they were hungry.

There is also mounting evidence that obesity is governed to some degree by variations in the human pool. In fact, recent studies have disclosed at least 30 new genes that may contribute to the onset of obesity and, in some cases, genes that may actually determine how fat will be distributed in an individual's body. For example, some individuals may collect fat predominantly in the abdomen and become "apple-shaped". Such individuals would be more likely to develop diabetes and heart disease. On the other hand, individuals whose distribution of fat predominates around the thighs and hips, or the so called "pear-shaped" individuals are less likely to develop diabetes and heart disease.

Yet another finding is that those who inherit the BMI–increasing DNA from their parents will weigh generally between 15 and 20 pounds more than normal individuals. This distinction is based solely upon genetic predisposition rather than lifestyle.

It is also interesting to note that, despite the broad prevalence of obesity worldwide, in recent years the rate of increase in this condition has actually begun to level off. In the U.S. the rate is actually beginning to show a decline, albeit, the U.S. is still among those nations having the highest rate of obesity, based primarily upon its industrial strength.

APPENDICES

Appendix I: *Glossary of Terms and Phrases*

* **Abdominoplasty:** also called a "tummy tuck". A procedure in which one or more incisions are made surgically in the lower abdomen to remove excess abdominal fat
* **Active Aggressive Lifestyle:** the lifestyle typical of athletes, military personnel and highly competitive individuals who exercise every day for more than two hours each day
* **Activity Metabolism Rate:** the rate at which calories are burned during daily activities, including exercise
* **Activity Metabolism:** making up 65% of total body metabolism, the calories burned for human functions such as heart beat, breathing and other normal life functions of the body
* **Acupuncture:** a controversial technique in which needles are strategically inserted into the skin along various parts of the body to stimulate neurological management of certain conditions, including obesity
* **Adenosine Triphosphate (ATP):** a chemical much like those in a simple flashlight battery that energizes human cellular function
* **Adipose Tissue:** body fat
* **Alimentary Canal:** the path that food takes through the human digestive system
* **Amino Acids:** the substance derived from proteins that is absorbed into the human blood stream for cell construction and repair
* **Amylase:** an enzyme contained in human saliva, and also secreted by the pancreas, that helps to break starches down into simple sugars called <u>glucose</u>
* **Anabolic Effect:** an increase in muscle and bone mass from exercise, steroid use or an increase in estrogen levels
* **Anorectic Agents:** drugs used to suppress appetite
* **Anorexia Nervosa:** a serious eating disorder characterized by severe malnutrition, physical wasting and starvation derived from a psychological abstention from eating regularly
* **Aspirator:** a vacuum device which draws fat through a hollow tube, called a <u>cannula</u>, in a lipoplasty or liposuction procedure
* **Bariatric Surgery:** the group of surgical procedures performed to either suppress appetite or interfere with normal nutrient absorption
* **Bile:** a digestive hormone produced in the liver which aids in the digestion of fats
* **Blood Sugar:** see <u>Glucose</u>
* **BMI Prime:** the percentage of body mass index to the upper limit of the normal range of BMI's (e.g., if the upper limit is 25 then a BMI of 22 yields a BMI Prime of 88%
* **Body Mass Index (BMI):** a broad measure of body mass equal to one's weight times 703 divided by the square of one's height

- **Bulimia Nervosa:** a serious eating disorder in which the victim interrupts long periods of fasting with intermittent eating binges and subsequent total purging by the induction of vomiting and/or precipitous use of laxatives
- **Caecum:** the junction at which the ileum enters into the large intestines
- **Calorie:** the term used to describe heat energy produced by human metabolism or the amount of heat energy required to raise the temperature of one gram of water one degree Celsius
- **Cannula:** a hollow tube attached to a suction device that used by plastic surgeons to remove excess fat in a lipoplasty or liposuction procedure
- **Capitation:** a type of healthcare insurance payment system by which a fixed periodic rate is paid under contract to a healthcare provider per enrolled patient or life
- **Carbohydrates:** the food nutrient or organic compound consisting of starches which are converted by digestive enzymes to glucose for energy metabolism
- **Cellulose:** the bulk, waxy substance of plants that is also known as fiber
- **Cholesterol:** a waxy metabolite derived from saturated animal fats, normal amounts of which are essential in producing digestive bile acids
- **Chyme:** the food contents of the stomach after having been broken down by digestive enzymes
- **Circadian Rhythm:** sometimes called the "human clock", a 24-cycle of biochemical, physiological and behavioral activities
- **Cortisol:** a hormone release by the adrenal gland during stress to increase blood sugar levels and appetite
- **Digestive Inhibitors:** drugs used to interfere with or interrupt the digestive process
- **Duodenum:** the upper end of the small intestines beginning at the pyloric sphincter, between the stomach and the jejunum
- **Elasticity of Demand:** a socioeconomic behavior that describes the degree by which individuals would alter their choice of one product for another
- **Endocannabinoid System (ECS):** a complex set of molecules in the central and peripheral nervous system that help to regulate and control pain, mood, appetite and memory
- **Epidemic:** the widespread prevalence of a contagious disease or condition not otherwise prevalent. See also Pandemic
- **Esophageal Sphincter:** the junction at which the esophagus enters the stomach
- **Esophagus:** the tube leading from the throat to the stomach
- **Ethnicity:** the term that distinguishes race by cultural origin
- **Fasting Plasma Glucose:** a test to determine the body's blood sugar levels after a period of fasting for usually as long as eight hours after a meal

- **Fat, Brown:** a type of adipose tissue found primarily in hibernating mammals and newborns, as well as small amounts in adults, that actually eats through white fat when activated by cold
- **Fat, Polyunsaturated:** a healthy, unsaturated oil derived from nuts, cheese (derivative), seeds, fish, algae and leafy greens
- **Fat, Saturated:** animal fat or lard
- **Fat, Unsaturated:** fat from vegetable oils
- **Fats:** the food nutrient which is converted by digestive enzymes to triglycerides for cell insulation and protection
- **Fiber:** a medium of non-digestible material having no calories that is passed through the digestive system as bulk
- **First-World:** a term used to describe highly developed and industrialized nations of the world
- **Gastrin:** the digestive hormone the stimulates the release of hydrochloric acid in the stomach to help digest into a substance called chyme
- **Ghrelin:** the hormone produced in the stomach and pancreas which induces the feeling of hunger
- **Glucose:** a simple sugar derived from the digestion of carbohydrate which is absorbed into the blood stream for energy metabolism
- **Glycemic Index:** a unit of measure which rates carbohydrates in terms of how quickly they are converted by digestive enzymes to glucose, the lower the value of this measure the slower will be the metabolism of carbohydrates
- **Glycogen:** a molecule made and stored primarily in the liver and muscles as an energy reserve because it can be quickly converted to glucose
- **Harris-Benedict Formula:** an equation used to measure required daily calorie consumption based on BMI and activity levels
- **Health Maintenance Organization (HMO):** a type of insurance plan in which patients are enrolled in an organization of employed providers
- **Hydrogenated Oils:** oils treated with the hydrogenation process
- **Hydrogenation:** the process of adding hydrogen to saturated and unsaturated oils in order to increase their shelf-life as well as their melting point
- **Hypercapnia:** a condition derived from too much carbon dioxide in the blood and can cause hyperventilation and death if prolonged
- **Hypercortisolism:** a condition derived from an overproduction of cortisol and is usually associated with Cushing's Disease
- **Hyperglycemia:** a condition in which blood sugar levels become elevated from insulin deficiency

- **Hypertension:** a serious condition derived from too much pressure against the walls of the blood vessels
- **Hypoglycemia:** a condition resulting from too little blood sugar derived from an overproduction of insulin
- **Hypoxia:** a condition derived from too little oxygen in the blood
- **Idiopathic Edema:** a condition having no definitive or specific cause in which fluid buildup around body tissue causes abnormal swelling
- **Ileum:** the distal or lower end of the small intestines, between the jejunum and caecum
- **Insulin Resistance:** the inability of the body to use insulin no matter how much is released by the pancreas
- **Insulin:** a digestive enzyme released by the pancreas to regulate the transfer of glucose into the blood stream
- **Jejunum:** the middle section of the small intestines, between the duodenum and ileum
- **Ketone:** an organic waste elevated during fasting as a substitute for energy
- **Ketosis:** a condition resulting from the accumulation of too much ketone waste
- **Kilocalorie:** the term often confused with calorie in that it should be used to describe calorie intake (i.e., a colloquially express "calorie" is actually a kilocalorie or 1,000 calories)
- **Kilogram:** 1,000 grams or the equivalent of 2.2 pounds
- **Leptin:** a protein hormone which helps to counteract neuropeptide Y in order to suppress appetite
- **Lipase:** the enzyme which breaks the fat into glycerol and fatty acids to produce triglycerides
- **Lipodissolve:** see Mesotherapy
- **Lipoplasty:** a group of cosmetic procedures performed to surgically remove body fat
- **Liposuction:** see Lipoplasty
- **Malabsorptive Bariatric Surgery (MBS):** a type of bariatric surgical procedure in various forms that performed to reduce the absorption of nutrients into the bloods stream usually by surgically by-passing portions of the small intestine
- **Mesotherapy:** a non-surgical cosmetic procedure in which certain chemicals are injected under the skin (subcutaneously) in order to dissolve away fat
- **Metabolic Syndrome:** a collection of events resulting usually from the effects of aging in which the body's metabolic rate begins to decline
- **Metabolism:** the organic process by which various chemicals, enzymes and hormones react to produce energy
- **Neuropeptide Y:** a neurotransmitter found in the brain and autonomic nervous system which regulates energy balance by regulating appetite and helping to increase the proportion of energy stored as fat

- **NHANES III:** a study of about 34,000 persons conducted between 1988 and 1994 from which a more accurate alternative to the Quetelet measure of body mass was derived
- **Obesity:** a potentially serious condition resulting from the accumulation of more than a normal amount of body fat
- **Pancreas:** the principal digestive endocrine gland which produces enzymes such as insulin and glucagon to help break down carbohydrates, proteins and fats into chyme
- **Pandemic:** a worldwide prevalence of a contagious disease or condition not otherwise prevalent
- **Passive-Aggressive Lifestyle:** an intermediate pattern of living engaged by most individuals who exercise at least three times per week for an hour each time
- **Passive-Sedentary Lifestyle:** the pattern of living engaged by individuals who exercise less than one hour per week or not at all
- **Peristalsis:** the wave-like action of digestive organs such as the esophagus to move food through the digestive process
- **Physiology:** the term used collectively to describe organic functions of the human body
- **Preferred Provider Organization (PPO):** a type of health insurance plan under which patients are enrolled in an organization of contract providers
- **Proteins:** the food nutrient which is converted by digestive enzymes to amino acids for cellular construction and repair
- **Pyloric Sphincter:** the junction at which the stomach is connected to the duodenum
- **Quetelet BMI:** see Body Mass Index
- **Race:** the term used to describe humans in accordance with their physical characteristics such as skin color, hair and facial features
- **Recommended Daily Allowance (RDA):** the minimum daily requirement for the essential nutrients, vitamins and minerals as published by the Food and Drug Administration
- **Restrictive Bariatric Surgery (RBS):** a type of bariatric surgical procedure in various forms that is performed to restrict the amount of food that can be consumed usually by reducing the size of the stomach
- **Rule of Ten's:** by this rule, in order to lose one pound in one year requires a reduction of 10 calories (kilocalories) per day
- **Satiety:** the feeling of fullness after eating a meal
- **Second- World:** a term used to describe largely agricultural and non-industrialized nations of the world
- **Seroma:** a subcutaneous (under the skin) pocket of fluids resulting often from a lipoplasty procedure
- **Thermic Effect of Food:** the process by which calories are burned to process fuel for energy

- **Thermic Metabolism Rate:** the rate used to describe the amount of calories (kilocalories) burned in the digestive process
- **Thermogenic Agents:** drugs used to increase thermic metabolism
- **Third-World:** a term used to describe largely impoverished and undeveloped nations of the world
- **Transfatty Acids:** a by-product of hydrogenated vegetable oils
- **Triglycerides:** a nutrient derived from fat that is absorbed into the blood stream to insulate and protect cells
- **Type 2 Diabetes:** a form of diabetes or <u>insulin</u> deficiency resulting from <u>insulin resistance</u>
- **Type A Personality:** a behavioral type characterized by aggressive, well-organized and highly competitive attributes
- **Type B Personality:** a behavioral type characterized by passive, laid-back and likable attributes
- **Universal Healthcare:** a national healthcare delivery system funded and administered by the federal government from tax revenues

Appendix II: *Table of Calories by Nutritional Content*

Adapted from the U.S. Department of Agriculture
National Nutrient Database, Release 17

Content Specified in Energy Calories (Kilocalories)
For Selected Foods in Alphabetical Order

Description	Weight (g)	Common Measure	Content per Measure
Alcoholic beverage, beer, light	354	12 fl oz	103
Alcoholic beverage, beer, regular	355	12 fl oz	138
Alcoholic beverage, daiquiri, prepared-from-recipe	60	2 fl oz	112
Alcoholic beverage, distilled, all (gin, rum, vodka, whiskey) 80 proof	42	1.5 fl oz	97
Alcoholic beverage, distilled, all (gin, rum, vodka, whiskey) 86 proof	42	1.5 fl oz	105
Alcoholic beverage, distilled, all (gin, rum, vodka, whiskey) 90 proof	42	1.5 fl oz	110
Alcoholic beverage, liqueur, coffee, 53 proof	52	1.5 fl oz	175
Alcoholic beverage, pina colada, prepared-from-recipe	141	4.5 fl oz	245
Alcoholic beverage, wine, dessert, dry	103	3.5 fl oz	157
Alcoholic beverage, wine, dessert, sweet	103	3.5 fl oz	165
Alcoholic beverage, wine, table, red	103	3.5 fl oz	74
Alcoholic beverage, wine, table, white	103	3.5 fl oz	70
Alfalfa seeds, sprouted, raw	33	1 cup	10
Apple juice, canned or bottled, unsweetened, without added ascorbic acid	248	1 cup	117
Apples, dried, sulfured, uncooked	32	5 rings	78
Apples, raw, with skin	138	1 apple	72
Apples, raw, without skin	110	1 cup	53
Applesauce, canned, sweetened, without salt	255	1 cup	194
Applesauce, canned, unsweetened, without added ascorbic acid	244	1 cup	105
Apricot nectar, canned, with added ascorbic acid	251	1 cup	141
Apricots, canned, heavy syrup pack, with skin, solids and liquids	258	1 cup	214
Apricots, canned, juice pack, with skin, solids and liquids	244	1 cup	117
Apricots, dried, sulfured, uncooked	35	10 halves	84
Apricots, raw	35	1 apricot	17
Artichokes, (globe or french), cooked, boiled, drained, without salt	168	1 cup	84
Artichokes, (globe or french), cooked, boiled, drained, without salt	120	1 medium	60
Asparagus, canned, drained solids	72	4 spears	14
Asparagus, cooked, boiled, drained	60	4 spears	13
Asparagus, frozen, cooked, boiled, drained, without salt	180	1 cup	32
Asparagus, frozen, cooked, boiled, drained, without salt	60	4 spears	11
Avocados, raw, California	28.35	1 oz	47
Avocados, raw, Florida	28.35	1 oz	34
Bagels, cinnamon-raisin	89	4" bagel	244
Bagels, cinnamon-raisin	71	3-1/2" bagel	195
Bagels, egg	89	4" bagel	247
Bagels, egg	71	3-1/2" bagel	197
Bagels, plain, enriched, with calcium propionate (includes onion, poppy, sesame)	71	3-1/2" bagel	195
Bagels, plain, enriched, with calcium propionate (includes onion, poppy, sesame)	89	4" bagel	245
Baking chocolate, unsweetened, liquid	28.35	1 oz	134
Baking chocolate, unsweetened, squares	28.35	1 square	142
Bamboo shoots, canned, drained solids	131	1 cup	25
Bananas, raw	118	1 banana	105
Bananas, raw	150	1 cup	134
Barley, pearled, cooked	157	1 cup	193
Barley, pearled, raw	200	1 cup	704
Beans, baked, canned, plain or vegetarian	254	1 cup	239

Description	Weight (g)	Common Measure	Content per Measure
Beans, baked, canned, with franks	259	1 cup	368
Beans, baked, canned, with pork and sweet sauce	253	1 cup	281
Beans, baked, canned, with pork and tomato sauce	253	1 cup	238
Beans, black, mature seeds, cooked, boiled, without salt	172	1 cup	227
Beans, great northern, mature seeds, cooked, boiled, without salt	177	1 cup	209
Beans, kidney, red, mature seeds, canned	256	1 cup	218
Beans, kidney, red, mature seeds, cooked, boiled, without salt	177	1 cup	225
Beans, navy, mature seeds, cooked, boiled, without salt	182	1 cup	255
Beans, pinto, mature seeds, cooked, boiled, without salt	171	1 cup	245
Beans, snap, green, canned, regular pack, drained solids	135	1 cup	27
Beans, snap, green, cooked, boiled, drained, without salt	125	1 cup	44
Beans, snap, green, frozen, cooked, boiled, drained without salt	135	1 cup	38
Beans, snap, yellow, canned, regular pack, drained solids	135	1 cup	27
Beans, snap, yellow, cooked, boiled, drained, without salt	125	1 cup	44
Beans, snap, yellow, frozen, cooked, boiled, drained, without salt	135	1 cup	38
Beans, white, mature seeds, canned	262	1 cup	307
Beef stew, canned entree	232	1 cup	218
Beef, chuck, blade roast, separable lean and fat, trimmed to 1/4" fat, all grades, cooked, braised	85	3 oz	293
Beef, chuck, blade roast, separable lean only, trimmed to 1/4" fat, all grades, cooked, braised	85	3 oz	213
Beef, cured, corned beef, canned	85.05	3 oz	213
Beef, cured, dried	28.35	1 oz	43
Beef, ground, 75% lean meat / 25% fat, patty, cooked, broiled	85	3 oz	236
Beef, ground, 80% lean meat / 20% fat, patty, cooked, broiled	85	3 oz	230
Beef, ground, 85% lean meat / 15% fat, patty, cooked, broiled	85	3 oz	213
Beef, rib, whole (ribs 6-12), separable lean and fat, trimmed to 1/4" fat, all grades, cooked, roasted	85	3 oz	304
Beef, rib, whole (ribs 6-12), separable lean only, trimmed to 1/4" fat, all grades, cooked, roasted	85	3 oz	195
Beef, round, bottom round, separable lean and fat, trimmed to 1/8" fat, all grades, cooked, braised	85	3 oz	210
Beef, round, bottom round, separable lean only, trimmed to 1/8" fat, all grades, cooked, braised	85	3 oz	184
Beef, round, eye of round, separable lean and fat, trimmed to 1/8" fat, all grades, cooked, roasted	85	3 oz	177
Beef, round, eye of round, separable lean only, trimmed to 1/8" fat, all grades, cooked, roasted	85	3 oz	144
Beef, top sirloin, separable lean and fat, trimmed to 1/8" fat, all grades, cooked, broiled	85	3 oz	207
Beef, top sirloin, separable lean only, trimmed to 1/8" fat, all grades, cooked, broiled	85	3 oz	151
Beef, variety meats and by-products, liver, cooked, pan-fried	85	3 oz	149
Beet greens, cooked, boiled, drained, without salt	144	1 cup	39
Beets, canned, drained solids	170	1 cup	53
Beets, canned, drained solids	24	1 beet	7
Beets, cooked, boiled, drained	50	1 beet	22
Beets, cooked, boiled, drained	170	1 cup	75
Biscuits, plain or buttermilk, prepared from recipe	101	4" biscuit	358
Biscuits, plain or buttermilk, prepared from recipe	60	2-1/2" biscuit	212
Biscuits, plain or buttermilk, refrigerated dough, higher fat, baked	27	2-1/2" biscuit	93
Biscuits, plain or buttermilk, refrigerated dough, lower fat, baked	21	2-1/4" biscuit	63
Blackberries, raw	144	1 cup	62

Description	Weight (g)	Common Measure	Content per Measure
Blueberries, frozen, sweetened	230	1 cup	186
Blueberries, raw	145	1 cup	83
Bologna, beef and pork	56.7	2 slices	175
Braunschweiger (a liver sausage), pork	56.7	2 slices	185
Bread crumbs, dry, grated, plain	28.35	1 oz	112
Bread crumbs, dry, grated, seasoned	120	1 cup	460
Bread stuffing, bread, dry mix, prepared	100	1/2 cup	178
Bread, banana, prepared from recipe, made with margarine	60	1 slice	196
Bread, cornbread, dry mix, prepared	60	1 piece	188
Bread, cornbread, prepared from recipe, made with low fat (2%) milk	65	1 piece	173
Bread, cracked-wheat	25	1 slice	65
Bread, egg	40	1/2" slice	115
Bread, french or vienna (includes sourdough)	25	1/2" slice	69
Bread, Indian, fry, made with lard (Navajo)	160	10-1/2" bread	528
Bread, Indian, fry, made with lard (Navajo)	90	5" bread	297
Bread, italian	20	1 slice	54
Bread, mixed-grain (includes whole-grain, 7-grain)	26	1 slice	65
Bread, mixed-grain, toasted (includes whole-grain, 7-grain)	24	1 slice	65
Bread, oatmeal	27	1 slice	73
Bread, oatmeal, toasted	25	1 slice	73
Bread, pita, white, enriched	28	4" pita	77
Bread, pita, white, enriched	60	6-1/2" pita	165
Bread, pumpernickel	32	1 slice	80
Bread, pumpernickel, toasted	29	1 slice	80
Bread, raisin, enriched	26	1 slice	71
Bread, raisin, toasted, enriched	24	1 slice	71
Bread, reduced-calorie, rye	23	1 slice	47
Bread, reduced-calorie, wheat	23	1 slice	46
Bread, reduced-calorie, white	23	1 slice	48
Bread, rye	32	1 slice	83
Bread, rye, toasted	24	1 slice	68
Bread, wheat (includes wheat berry)	25	1 slice	65
Bread, wheat, toasted (includes wheat berry)	23	1 slice	65
Bread, white, commercially prepared (includes soft bread crumbs)	25	1 slice	67
Bread, white, commercially prepared (includes soft bread crumbs)	45	1 cup	120
Bread, white, commercially prepared, toasted	22	1 slice	64
Bread, whole-wheat, commercially prepared	28	1 slice	69
Bread, whole-wheat, commercially prepared, toasted	25	1 slice	69
Breakfast items, biscuit with egg and sausage	180	1 biscuit	581
Breakfast items, french toast with butter	135	2 slices	356
Broccoli, cooked, boiled, drained, without salt	156	1 cup	55
Broccoli, cooked, boiled, drained, without salt	37	1 spear	13
Broccoli, flower clusters, raw	11	1 floweret	3
Broccoli, frozen, chopped, cooked, boiled, drained, without salt	184	1 cup	52
Broccoli, raw	31	1 spear	11
Broccoli, raw	88	1 cup	30
Brussels sprouts, cooked, boiled, drained, without salt	156	1 cup	56
Brussels sprouts, frozen, cooked, boiled, drained, without salt	155	1 cup	65

Description	Weight (g)	Common Measure	Content per Measure
Buckwheat flour, whole-groat	120	1 cup	402
Buckwheat groats, roasted, cooked	168	1 cup	155
Bulgur, cooked	182	1 cup	151
Bulgur, dry	140	1 cup	479
Butter, salted	14.2	1 tbsp	102
Butter, without salt	14.2	1 tbsp	102
Cabbage, chinese (pak-choi), cooked, boiled, drained, without salt	170	1 cup	20
Cabbage, chinese (pe-tsai), cooked, boiled, drained, without salt	119	1 cup	17
Cabbage, cooked, boiled, drained, without salt	150	1 cup	33
Cabbage, raw	70	1 cup	17
Cabbage, red, raw	70	1 cup	22
Cabbage, savoy, raw	70	1 cup	19
Cake, angelfood, commercially prepared	28	1 piece	72
Cake, angelfood, dry mix, prepared	50	1 piece	129
Cake, boston cream pie, commercially prepared	92	1 piece	232
Cake, chocolate, commercially prepared with chocolate frosting	64	1 piece	235
Cake, chocolate, prepared from recipe without frosting	95	1 piece	340
Cake, fruitcake, commercially prepared	43	1 piece	139
Cake, gingerbread, prepared from recipe	74	1 piece	263
Cake, pineapple upside-down, prepared from recipe	115	1 piece	367
Cake, pound, commercially prepared, butter	28	1 piece	109
Cake, pound, commercially prepared, fat-free	28	1 slice	79
Cake, shortcake, biscuit-type, prepared from recipe	65	1 shortcake	225
Cake, snack cakes, creme-filled, chocolate with frosting	50	1 cupcake	188
Cake, snack cakes, creme-filled, sponge	42.5	1 cake	155
Cake, snack cakes, cupcakes, chocolate, with frosting, low-fat	43	1 cupcake	131
Cake, sponge, commercially prepared	30	1 shortcake	87
Cake, sponge, prepared from recipe	63	1 piece	187
Cake, white, prepared from recipe with coconut frosting	112	1 piece	399
Cake, white, prepared from recipe without frosting	74	1 piece	264
Cake, yellow, commercially prepared, with chocolate frosting	64	1 piece	243
Cake, yellow, commercially prepared, with vanilla frosting	64	1 piece	239
Candies, caramels	10.1	1 piece	39
Candies, caramels, chocolate-flavor roll	7	1 piece	27
Candies, carob	28.35	1 oz	153
Candies, confectioner's coating, white	170	1 cup	916
Candies, fudge, chocolate, prepared-from-recipe	17	1 piece	70
Candies, fudge, chocolate, with nuts, prepared-from-recipe	19	1 piece	88
Candies, fudge, vanilla with nuts	15	1 piece	65
Candies, fudge, vanilla, prepared-from-recipe	16	1 piece	61
Candies, gumdrops, starch jelly pieces	22	10 bears	87
Candies, gumdrops, starch jelly pieces	74	10 worms	293
Candies, gumdrops, starch jelly pieces	4.2	1 medium	17
Candies, hard	3	1 small piece	12
Candies, hard	6	1 piece	24
Candies, jellybeans	28.35	10 large	106
Candies, KITKAT Wafer Bar	42	1 bar (1.5 oz)	218
Candies, M&MMARS, "M&M's" Milk Chocolate Candies	7	10 pieces	34

Description	Weight (g)	Common Measure	Content per Measure
Candies, M&M MARS, "M&M's" Peanut Chocolate Candies	20	10 pieces	103
Candies, M&M MARS, MARS MILKY WAY Bar	61	1 bar (2.15 oz)	258
Candies, M&M MARS, MARS MILKY WAY Bar	18	1 fun size bar	76
Candies, M&M MARS, SNICKERS Bar	57	1 bar (2 oz)	266
Candies, M&M MARS, STARBURST Fruit Chews	5	1 piece	20
Candies, marshmallows	50	1 cup	159
Candies, milk chocolate	44	1 bar (1.55 oz)	235
Candies, milk chocolate coated peanuts	40	10 pieces	208
Candies, milk chocolate coated raisins	10	10 pieces	39
Candies, milk chocolate, with almonds	41	1 bar (1.45 oz)	216
Candies, MR. GOODBAR Chocolate Bar	49	1 bar (1.75 oz)	264
Candies, NESTLE, BUTTERFINGER Bar	7	1 fun size bar	33
Candies, NESTLE, CRUNCH Bar and Dessert Topping	44	1 bar (1.55 oz)	230
Candies, REESE'S Peanut Butter Cups	45	1 package (contains 2)	232
Candies, semisweet chocolate	168	1 cup	805
Candies, SPECIAL DARK Chocolate Bar	8.4	1 miniature	45
Carambola, (starfruit), raw	108	1 cup	33
Carambola, (starfruit), raw	91	1 fruit	28
Carbonated beverage, club soda	355	12 fl oz	0
Carbonated beverage, cola, contains caffeine	370	12 fl oz	155
Carbonated beverage, ginger ale	366	12 fl oz	124
Carbonated beverage, grape soda	372	12 fl oz	160
Carbonated beverage, lemon-lime soda	368	12 fl oz	147
Carbonated beverage, low calorie, cola or pepper-type, with aspartame, contains caffeine	355	12 fl oz	4
Carbonated beverage, low calorie, other than cola or pepper, without caffeine	355	12 fl oz	0
Carbonated beverage, orange	372	12 fl oz	179
Carbonated beverage, pepper-type, contains caffeine	368	12 fl oz	151
Carbonated beverage, root beer	370	12 fl oz	152
Carob flour	8	1 tbsp	18
Carrot juice, canned	236	1 cup	94
Carrots, baby, raw	10	1 medium	4
Carrots, canned, regular pack, drained solids	146	1 cup	37
Carrots, cooked, boiled, drained, without salt	156	1 cup	55
Carrots, frozen, cooked, boiled, drained, without salt	146	1 cup	54
Carrots, raw	110	1 cup	45
Carrots, raw	72	1 carrot	30
Catsup	6	1 packet	6
Catsup	15	1 tbsp	15
Cauliflower, cooked, boiled, drained, without salt	124	1 cup	29
Cauliflower, cooked, boiled, drained, without salt	54	3 flowerets	12
Cauliflower, frozen, cooked, boiled, drained, without salt	180	1 cup	34
Cauliflower, raw	13	1 floweret	3
Cauliflower, raw	100	1 cup	25
Celery, cooked, boiled, drained, without salt	37.5	1 stalk	7
Celery, cooked, boiled, drained, without salt	150	1 cup	27
Celery, raw	40	1 stalk	6
Celery, raw	120	1 cup	17

Description	Weight (g)	Common Measure	Content per Measure
Cereals ready-to-eat, GENERAL MILLS, APPLE CINNAMON CHEERIOS	30	3/4 cup	118
Cereals ready-to-eat, GENERAL MILLS, BASIC 4	55	1 cup	202
Cereals ready-to-eat, GENERAL MILLS, BERRY BERRY KIX	30	3/4 cup	118
Cereals ready-to-eat, GENERAL MILLS, CHEERIOS	30	1 cup	111
Cereals ready-to-eat, GENERAL MILLS, CINNAMON TOAST CRUNCH	30	3/4 cup	127
Cereals ready-to-eat, GENERAL MILLS, COCOA PUFFS	30	1 cup	117
Cereals ready-to-eat, GENERAL MILLS, Corn CHEX	30	1 cup	112
Cereals ready-to-eat, GENERAL MILLS, FROSTED WHEATIES	30	3/4 cup	112
Cereals ready-to-eat, GENERAL MILLS, GOLDEN GRAHAMS	30	3/4 cup	112
Cereals ready-to-eat, GENERAL MILLS, HONEY NUT CHEERIOS	30	1 cup	112
Cereals ready-to-eat, GENERAL MILLS, Honey Nut CHEX	30	3/4 cup	114
Cereals ready-to-eat, GENERAL MILLS, HONEY NUT CLUSTERS	55	1 cup	214
Cereals ready-to-eat, GENERAL MILLS, KIX	30	1-1/3 cup	115
Cereals ready-to-eat, GENERAL MILLS, LUCKY CHARMS	30	1 cup	114
Cereals ready-to-eat, GENERAL MILLS, RAISIN NUT BRAN	55	1 cup	209
Cereals ready-to-eat, GENERAL MILLS, REESE'S PUFFS	30	3/4 cup	128
Cereals ready-to-eat, GENERAL MILLS, Rice CHEX	31	1-1/4 cup	117
Cereals ready-to-eat, GENERAL MILLS, TOTAL Corn Flakes	30	1-1/3 cup	112
Cereals ready-to-eat, GENERAL MILLS, TOTAL Raisin Bran	55	1 cup	171
Cereals ready-to-eat, GENERAL MILLS, TRIX	30	1 cup	117
Cereals ready-to-eat, GENERAL MILLS, Wheat CHEX	30	1 cup	104
Cereals ready-to-eat, GENERAL MILLS, WHEATIES	30	1 cup	107
Cereals ready-to-eat, GENERAL MILLS, Whole Grain TOTAL	30	3/4 cup	97
Cereals ready-to-eat, KELLOGG, KELLOGG'S ALL-BRAN Original	30	1/2 cup	78
Cereals ready-to-eat, KELLOGG, KELLOGG'S APPLE JACKS	30	1 cup	117
Cereals ready-to-eat, KELLOGG, KELLOGG'S COCOA KRISPIES	31	3/4 cup	118
Cereals ready-to-eat, KELLOGG, KELLOGG'S Complete Wheat Bran Flakes	29	3/4 cup	92
Cereals ready-to-eat, KELLOGG, KELLOGG'S Corn Flakes	28	1 cup	101
Cereals ready-to-eat, KELLOGG, KELLOGG'S CORN POPS	31	1 cup	118
Cereals ready-to-eat, KELLOGG, KELLOGG'S CRISPIX	29	1 cup	109
Cereals ready-to-eat, KELLOGG, KELLOGG'S FROOT LOOPS	30	1 cup	118
Cereals ready-to-eat, KELLOGG, KELLOGG'S FROSTED FLAKES	31	3/4 cup	114
Cereals ready-to-eat, KELLOGG, KELLOGG'S FROSTED MINI-WHEATS, bite size	55	1 cup	189
Cereals ready-to-eat, KELLOGG, KELLOGG'S PRODUCT 19	30	1 cup	100
Cereals ready-to-eat, KELLOGG, KELLOGG'S RAISIN BRAN	61	1 cup	195
Cereals ready-to-eat, KELLOGG, KELLOGG'S RICE KRISPIES	33	1-1/4 cup	119
Cereals ready-to-eat, KELLOGG, KELLOGG'S RICE KRISPIES TREATS Cereal	30	3/4 cup	122
Cereals ready-to-eat, KELLOGG, KELLOGG'S SMACKS	27	3/4 cup	104
Cereals ready-to-eat, KELLOGG, KELLOGG'S SPECIAL K	31	1 cup	117
Cereals ready-to-eat, KELLOGG'S FROSTED MINI-WHEATS, original	51	1 cup	175
Cereals ready-to-eat, QUAKER, CAP'N CRUNCH	27	3/4 cup	108
Cereals ready-to-eat, QUAKER, CAP'N CRUNCH with CRUNCHBERRIES	26	3/4 cup	104
Cereals ready-to-eat, QUAKER, CAP'N CRUNCH'S PEANUT BUTTER CRUNCH	27	3/4 cup	112
Cereals ready-to-eat, QUAKER, Honey Nut Heaven	49	1 cup	192

Description	Weight (g)	Common Measure	Content per Measure
Cereals ready-to-eat, QUAKER, Low Fat 100% Natural Granola with Raisins	50	1/2 cup	195
Cereals ready-to-eat, QUAKER, QUAKER 100% Natural Cereal with oats, honey, and raisins	51	1/2 cup	237
Cereals ready-to-eat, QUAKER, QUAKER OAT CINNAMON LIFE	32	3/4 cup	120
Cereals ready-to-eat, QUAKER, QUAKER OAT LIFE, plain	32	3/4 cup	120
Cereals ready-to-eat, rice, puffed, fortified	14	1 cup	56
Cereals ready-to-eat, wheat germ, toasted, plain	7.119	1 tbsp	27
Cereals ready-to-eat, wheat, puffed, fortified	12	1 cup	44
Cereals ready-to-eat, wheat, shredded, plain, sugar and salt free	46	2 biscuits	155
Cereals, corn grits, white, regular and quick, enriched, cooked with water, without salt	242	1 cup	143
Cereals, corn grits, yellow, regular and quick, enriched, cooked with water, without salt	242	1 cup	143
Cereals, CREAM OF WHEAT, mix'n eat, plain, prepared with water	142	1 packet	102
Cereals, CREAM OF WHEAT, quick, cooked with water, without salt	239	1 cup	129
Cereals, CREAM OF WHEAT, regular, cooked with water, without salt	251	1 cup	126
Cereals, MALT-O-MEAL, plain and chocolate, cooked with water, without salt	240	1 cup	122
Cereals, oats, instant, fortified, plain, prepared with water	177	1 packet	97
Cereals, oats, regular and quick and instant, unenriched, cooked with water, without salt	234	1 cup	147
Cereals, QUAKER, corn grits, instant, plain, prepared with water	137	1 packet	93
Cereals, QUAKER, Instant Oatmeal, maple and brown sugar, prepared with boiling water	155	1 packet	157
Cereals, QUAKER, Instant Oatmeal, apples and cinnamon, prepared with boiling water	149	1 packet	130
Cereals, WHEATENA, cooked with water	243	1 cup	136
Cheese food, pasteurized process, american, without di sodium phosphate	28.35	1 oz	94
Cheese sauce, prepared from recipe	243	1 cup	479
Cheese spread, pasteurized process, american, without di sodium phosphate	28.35	1 oz	82
Cheese, blue	28.35	1 oz	100
Cheese, camembert	38	1 wedge	114
Cheese, cheddar	28.35	1 oz	114
Cheese, cottage, creamed, large or small curd	210	1 cup	216
Cheese, cottage, creamed, with fruit	226	1 cup	219
Cheese, cottage, lowfat, 1% milkfat	226	1 cup	163
Cheese, cottage, lowfat, 2% milkfat	226	1 cup	203
Cheese, cottage, nonfat, uncreamed, dry, large or small curd	145	1 cup	123
Cheese, cream	14.5	1 tbsp	51
Cheese, cream, fat free	15.6	1 tbsp	15
Cheese, feta	28.35	1 oz	75
Cheese, low fat, cheddar or colby	28.35	1 oz	49
Cheese, mozzarella, part skim milk, low moisture	28.35	1 oz	86
Cheese, mozzarella, whole milk	28.35	1 oz	85
Cheese, muenster	28.35	1 oz	104
Cheese, neufchatel	28.35	1 oz	74
Cheese, parmesan, grated	5	1 tbsp	22
Cheese, pasteurized process, american, with di sodium phosphate	28.35	1 oz	106
Cheese, pasteurized process, swiss, with di sodium phosphate	28.35	1 oz	95

Description	Weight (g)	Common Measure	Content per Measure
Cheese, provolone	28.35	1 oz	100
Cheese, ricotta, part skim milk	246	1 cup	339
Cheese, ricotta, whole milk	246	1 cup	428
Cheese, swiss	28.35	1 oz	108
Cheesecake commercially prepared	80	1 piece	257
Cherries, sour, red, canned, water pack, solids and liquids (includes USDA commodity red tart cherries, canned)	244	1 cup	88
Cherries, sweet, raw	68	10 cherries	43
Chicken pot pie, frozen entree	217	1 small pie	484
Chicken roll, light meat	56.7	2 slices	87
Chicken, broilers or fryers, breast, meat and skin, cooked, fried, batter	140	1/2 breast	364
Chicken, broilers or fryers, breast, meat and skin, cooked, fried, flour	98	1/2 breast	218
Chicken, broilers or fryers, breast, meat only, cooked, roasted	86	1/2 breast	142
Chicken, broilers or fryers, dark meat, meat only, cooked, fried	84	3 oz	203
Chicken, broilers or fryers, drumstick, meat and skin, cooked, fried, batter	72	1 drumstick	193
Chicken, broilers or fryers, drumstick, meat and skin, cooked, fried, flour	49	1 drumstick	120
Chicken, broilers or fryers, drumstick, meat only, cooked, roasted	44	1 drumstick	76
Chicken, broilers or fryers, giblets, cooked, simmered	145	1 cup	229
Chicken, broilers or fryers, light meat, meat only, cooked, fried	84	3 oz	181
Chicken, broilers or fryers, neck, meat only, cooked, simmered	18	1 neck	32
Chicken, broilers or fryers, thigh, meat and skin, cooked, fried, batter	86	1 thigh	238
Chicken, broilers or fryers, thigh, meat only, cooked, roasted	52	1 thigh	109
Chicken, broilers or fryers, wing, meat and skin, cooked, fried, batter	49	1 wing	159
Chicken, canned, meat only, with broth	142	5 oz	234
Chicken, liver, all classes, cooked, simmered	19.6	1 liver	33
Chicken, stewing, meat only, cooked, stewed	140	1 cup	332
Chickpeas (garbanzo beans, bengal gram), mature seeds, canned	240	1 cup	286
Chickpeas (garbanzo beans, bengal gram), mature seeds, cooked, boiled, without salt	164	1 cup	269
Chili con carne with beans, canned entree	222	1 cup	289
Chives, raw	3	1 tbsp	1
Chocolate syrup	18.75	1 tbsp	52
Chocolate-flavor beverage mix for milk, powder, without added nutrients	21.6	2-3 heaping tsp	75
Chocolate-flavor beverage mix, powder, prepared with whole milk	266	1 cup	226
Cocoa mix, no sugar added, powder	15	1/2 oz envelope	56
Cocoa mix, powder	28.35	3 heaping tsp	113
Cocoa mix, powder, prepared with water	206	1 serving	113
Cocoa mix, with aspartame, powder, prepared from item 14196	192	1 serving	56
Cocoa, dry powder, unsweetened	5.4	1 tbsp	12
Coffee, brewed from grounds, prepared with tap water	178	6 fl oz	2
Coffee, brewed, espresso, restaurant-prepared	60	2 fl oz	1
Coffee, instant, regular, prepared with water	179	6 fl oz	4
Coffeecake, cinnamon with crumb topping, commercially prepared, enriched	63	1 piece	263
Coleslaw, home-prepared	120	1 cup	83
Collards, cooked, boiled, drained, without salt	190	1 cup	49
Collards, frozen, chopped, cooked, boiled, drained, without salt	170	1 cup	61
Cookies, brownies, commercially prepared	56	1 brownie	227

Description	Weight (g)	Common Measure	Content per Measure
Cookies, brownies, dry mix, special dietary, prepared	22	1 brownie	84
Cookies, butter, commercially prepared, enriched	5	1 cookie	23
Cookies, chocolate chip, commercially prepared, reg, higher fat, enriched	10	1 cookie	49
Cookies, chocolate chip, commercially prepared, regular, lower fat	10	1 cookie	45
Cookies, chocolate chip, prepared from recipe, made with margarine	16	1 cookie	78
Cookies, chocolate chip, refrigerated dough, baked	26	1 cookie	128
Cookies, chocolate sandwich, with creme filling, regular	10	1 cookie	47
Cookies, fig bars	16	1 cookie	56
Cookies, graham crackers, plain or honey (includes cinnamon)	14	2 squares	59
Cookies, graham crackers, plain or honey (includes cinnamon)	84	1 cup	355
Cookies, molasses	15	1 cookie, medium	65
Cookies, molasses	32	1 cookie, large (3-1/2" to 4")	138
Cookies, oatmeal, commercially prepared, fat-free	11	1 cookie	36
Cookies, oatmeal, commercially prepared, regular	25	1 cookie	113
Cookies, oatmeal, commercially prepared, soft-type	15	1 cookie	61
Cookies, oatmeal, prepared from recipe, with raisins	15	1 cookie	65
Cookies, peanut butter, commercially prepared, regular	15	1 cookie	72
Cookies, peanut butter, prepared from recipe	20	1 cookie	95
Cookies, shortbread, commercially prepared, pecan	14	1 cookie	76
Cookies, shortbread, commercially prepared, plain	8	1 cookie	40
Cookies, sugar, commercially prepared, regular (includes vanilla)	15	1 cookie	72
Cookies, sugar, prepared from recipe, made with margarine	14	1 cookie	66
Cookies, sugar, refrigerated dough, baked	15	1 cookie	73
Cookies, vanilla sandwich with creme filling	10	1 cookie	48
Cookies, vanilla sandwich with creme filling	15	1 cookie	72
Cookies, vanilla wafers, lower fat	4	1 cookie	18
Corn, sweet, white, cooked, boiled, drained, without salt	77	1 ear	83
Corn, sweet, yellow, canned, cream style, regular pack	256	1 cup	184
Corn, sweet, yellow, canned, vacuum pack, regular pack	210	1 cup	166
Corn, sweet, yellow, cooked, boiled, drained, without salt	77	1 ear	83
Corn, sweet, yellow, frozen, kernels cut off cob, boiled, drained, without salt	164	1 cup	133
Corn, sweet, yellow, frozen, kernels on cob, cooked, boiled, drained, without salt	63	1 ear	59
Cornmeal, degermed, enriched, yellow	138	1 cup	505
Cornmeal, self-rising, degermed, enriched, yellow	138	1 cup	490
Cornmeal, whole-grain, yellow	122	1 cup	442
Cornstarch	8.064	1 tbsp	31
Couscous, cooked	157	1 cup	176
Couscous, dry	173	1 cup	650
Cowpeas (Blackeyes), immature seeds, cooked, boiled, drained, without salt	165	1 cup	160
Cowpeas (blackeyes), immature seeds, frozen, cooked, boiled, drained, without salt	170	1 cup	224
Cowpeas, common (blackeyes, crowder, southern), mature seeds, canned, plain	240	1 cup	185
Cowpeas, common (blackeyes, crowder, southern), mature seeds, cooked, boiled, without salt	172	1 cup	200
Crackers, cheese, regular	10	10 crackers	50
Crackers, cheese, sandwich-type with peanut butter filling	7	1 sandwich	35

Description	Weight (g)	Common Measure	Content per Measure
Crackers, matzo, plain	28.35	1 matzo	112
Crackers, melba toast, plain	20	4 pieces	78
Crackers, rye, wafers, plain	11	1 wafer	37
Crackers, saltines (includes oyster, soda, soup)	12	4 crackers	51
Crackers, standard snack-type, regular	12	4 crackers	60
Crackers, standard snack-type, sandwich, with cheese filling	7	1 sandwich	33
Crackers, wheat, regular	8	4 crackers	38
Crackers, whole-wheat	16	4 crackers	71
Cranberry juice cocktail, bottled	253	8 fl oz	144
Cranberry sauce, canned, sweetened	57	1 slice	86
Cream substitute, liquid, with hydrogenated vegetable oil and soy protein	15	1 tbsp	20
Cream substitute, powdered	2	1 tsp	11
Cream, fluid, half and half	15	1 tbsp	20
Cream, fluid, heavy whipping	15	1 tbsp	52
Cream, fluid, light (coffee cream or table cream)	15	1 tbsp	29
Cream, fluid, light whipping	15	1 tbsp	44
Cream, sour, cultured	12	1 tbsp	26
Cream, sour, reduced fat, cultured	15	1 tbsp	20
Cream, whipped, cream topping, pressurized	3	1 tbsp	8
Croissants, butter	57	1 croissant	231
Croutons, seasoned	40	1 cup	186
Crustaceans, crab, alaska king, cooked, moist heat	85	3 oz	82
Crustaceans, crab, alaska king, imitation, made from surimi	85	3 oz	87
Crustaceans, crab, blue, canned	135	1 cup	134
Crustaceans, crab, blue, cooked, moist heat	85	3 oz	87
Crustaceans, crab, blue, crab cakes	60	1 cake	93
Crustaceans, lobster, northern, cooked, moist heat	85	3 oz	83
Crustaceans, shrimp, mixed species, canned	85.05	3 oz	102
Crustaceans, shrimp, mixed species, cooked, breaded and fried	45	6 large	109
Crustaceans, shrimp, mixed species, cooked, breaded and fried	85	3 oz	206
Cucumber, peeled, raw	119	1 cup	14
Cucumber, peeled, raw	280	1 large	34
Cucumber, with peel, raw	301	1 large	45
Cucumber, with peel, raw	104	1 cup	16
Dandelion greens, cooked, boiled, drained, without salt	105	1 cup	35
Danish pastry, cheese	71	1 danish	266
Danish pastry, fruit, enriched (includes apple, cinnamon, raisin, lemon, raspberry, strawberry)	71	1 danish	263
Dates, deglet noor	178	1 cup	502
Dates, deglet noor	41.5	5 dates	117
Dessert topping, powdered, 1.5 ounce prepared with 1/2 cup milk	4	1 tbsp	8
Dessert topping, pressurized	4	1 tbsp	11
Dessert topping, semi solid, frozen	4	1 tbsp	13
Dill weed, fresh	1	5 sprigs	0
Doughnuts, cake-type, plain (includes unsugared, old-fashioned)	14	1 hole	59
Doughnuts, cake-type, plain (includes unsugared, old-fashioned)	47	1 medium	198
Doughnuts, yeast-leavened, glazed, enriched (includes honey buns)	13	1 hole	52
Doughnuts, yeast-leavened, glazed, enriched (includes honey buns)	60	1 medium	242

Description	Weight (g)	Common Measure	Content per Measure
Duck, domesticated, meat only, cooked, roasted	221	1/2 duck	444
Eclairs, custard-filled with chocolate glaze, prepared from recipe	100	1 eclair	262
Egg substitute, liquid	62.75	1/4 cup	53
Egg, white, raw, fresh	33.4	1 large	17
Egg, whole, cooked, fried	46	1 large	92
Egg, whole, cooked, hard-boiled	50	1 large	78
Egg, whole, cooked, poached	50	1 large	74
Egg, whole, cooked, scrambled	61	1 large	101
Egg, whole, raw, fresh	44	1 medium	65
Egg, whole, raw, fresh	50	1 large	74
Egg, whole, raw, fresh	58	1 extra large	85
Egg, yolk, raw, fresh	16.6	1 large	53
Eggnog	254	1 cup	343
Eggplant, cooked, boiled, drained, without salt	99	1 cup	35
Endive, raw	50	1 cup	9
English muffins, plain, enriched, with ca prop (includes sourdough)	57	1 muffin	134
English muffins, plain, toasted, enriched, with calcium propionate (includes sourdough)	52	1 muffin	133
Entrees, fish fillet, battered or breaded, and fried	91	1 fillet	211
Entrees, pizza with pepperoni	71	1 slice	181
Fast foods, burrito, with beans and cheese	93	1 burrito	189
Fast foods, burrito, with beans and meat	115.5	1 burrito	254
Fast foods, cheeseburger, large, single patty, with condiments and vegetables	219	1 sandwich	563
Fast foods, cheeseburger, regular, double patty and bun, plain	160	1 sandwich	461
Fast foods, cheeseburger, regular, double patty, plain	155	1 sandwich	457
Fast foods, cheeseburger, regular, double patty, with condiments and vegetables	166	1 sandwich	417
Fast foods, cheeseburger, regular, single patty, with condiments	113	1 sandwich	295
Fast foods, chicken fillet sandwich, plain	182	1 sandwich	515
Fast foods, chicken, breaded and fried, boneless pieces, plain	106	6 pieces	315
Fast foods, chili con carne	253	1 cup	256
Fast foods, chimichanga, with beef	174	1 chimichanga	425
Fast foods, clams, breaded and fried	115	3/4 cup	451
Fast foods, coleslaw	99	3/4 cup	147
Fast foods, croissant, with egg, cheese, and bacon	129	1 croissant	413
Fast foods, danish pastry, cheese	91	1 pastry	353
Fast foods, danish pastry, fruit	94	1 pastry	335
Fast foods, enchilada, with cheese	163	1 enchilada	319
Fast foods, english muffin, with egg, cheese, and canadian bacon	137	1 muffin	289
Fast foods, fish sandwich, with tartar sauce and cheese	183	1 sandwich	523
Fast foods, french toast sticks	141	5 sticks	513
Fast foods, frijoles with cheese	167	1 cup	225
Fast foods, hamburger, large, double patty, with condiments and vegetables	226	1 sandwich	540
Fast foods, hamburger, regular, double patty, with condiments	215	1 sandwich	576
Fast foods, hamburger, regular, single patty, with condiments	106	1 sandwich	272
Fast foods, hotdog, plain	98	1 sandwich	242
Fast foods, hotdog, with chili	114	1 sandwich	296
Fast foods, hotdog, with corn flour coating (corndog)	175	1 corn dog	460

Description	Weight (g)	Common Measure	Content per Measure
Fast foods, hush puppies	78	5 pieces	257
Fast foods, ice milk, vanilla, soft-serve, with cone	103	1 cone	164
Fast foods, nachos, with cheese	113	6-8 nachos	346
Fast foods, onion rings, breaded and fried	83	8-9 rings	276
Fast foods, pancakes with butter and syrup	232	2 pancakes	520
Fast foods, potato, french fried in vegetable oil	169	1 large	578
Fast foods, potato, french fried in vegetable oil	134	1 medium	458
Fast foods, potato, french fried in vegetable oil	85	1 small	291
Fast foods, potato, mashed	80	1/3 cup	66
Fast foods, potatoes, hashed brown	72	1/2 cup	151
Fast foods, roast beef sandwich, plain	139	1 sandwich	346
Fast foods, salad, vegetable, tossed, without dressing, with cheese and egg	217	1-1/2 cups	102
Fast foods, salad, vegetable, tossed, without dressing, with chicken	218	1-1/2 cups	105
Fast foods, shrimp, breaded and fried	164	6-8 shrimp	454
Fast foods, submarine sandwich, with cold cuts	228	1 sandwich, 6" roll	456
Fast foods, submarine sandwich, with roast beef	216	1 sandwich, 6" roll	410
Fast foods, submarine sandwich, with tuna salad	256	1 sandwich, 6" roll	584
Fast foods, sundae, hot fudge	158	1 sundae	284
Fast foods, taco	263	1 large	568
Fast foods, taco	171	1 small	369
Fast foods, taco salad	198	1-1/2 cups	279
Fast foods, tostada, with beans, beef, and cheese	225	1 tostada	333
Figs, dried, uncooked	38	2 figs	95
Fish, catfish, channel, cooked, breaded and fried	85	3 oz	195
Fish, cod, Atlantic, canned, solids and liquid	85	3 oz	89
Fish, cod, Pacific, cooked, dry heat	85	3 oz	89
Fish, fish portions and sticks, frozen, preheated	57	1 portion (4" x 2" x 1/2")	155
Fish, fish portions and sticks, frozen, preheated	28	1 stick (4" x 1" x 1/2")	76
Fish, flatfish (flounder and sole species), cooked, dry heat	127	1 fillet	149
Fish, flatfish (flounder and sole species), cooked, dry heat	85	3 oz	99
Fish, haddock, cooked, dry heat	85	3 oz	95
Fish, haddock, cooked, dry heat	150	1 fillet	168
Fish, halibut, Atlantic and Pacific, cooked, dry heat	159	1/2 fillet	223
Fish, halibut, Atlantic and Pacific, cooked, dry heat	85	3 oz	119
Fish, herring, Atlantic, pickled	85.05	3 oz	223
Fish, ocean perch, Atlantic, cooked, dry heat	50	1 fillet	61
Fish, ocean perch, Atlantic, cooked, dry heat	85	3 oz	103
Fish, pollock, walleye, cooked, dry heat	60	1 fillet	68
Fish, pollock, walleye, cooked, dry heat	85	3 oz	96
Fish, rockfish, Pacific, mixed species, cooked, dry heat	149	1 fillet	180
Fish, rockfish, Pacific, mixed species, cooked, dry heat	85	3 oz	103
Fish, roughy, orange, cooked, dry heat	85	3 oz	76
Fish, salmon, chinook, smoked	85.05	3 oz	100
Fish, salmon, pink, canned, solids with bone and liquid	85	3 oz	118
Fish, salmon, sockeye, cooked, dry heat	155	1/2 fillet	335
Fish, salmon, sockeye, cooked, dry heat	85	3 oz	184
Fish, sardine, Atlantic, canned in oil, drained solids with bone	85.05	3 oz	177
Fish, swordfish, cooked, dry heat	85	3 oz	132

Description	Weight (g)	Common Measure	Content per Measure
Fish, swordfish, cooked, dry heat	106	1 piece	164
Fish, trout, rainbow, farmed, cooked, dry heat	85	3 oz	144
Fish, tuna salad	205	1 cup	383
Fish, tuna, light, canned in oil, drained solids	85.05	3 oz	168
Fish, tuna, light, canned in water, drained solids	85	3 oz	99
Fish, tuna, white, canned in water, drained solids	85	3 oz	109
Fish, tuna, yellowfin, fresh, cooked, dry heat	85	3 oz	118
Frankfurter, beef	45	1 frank	149
Frankfurter, beef and pork	45	1 frank	137
Frankfurter, chicken	45	1 frank	116
French toast, frozen, ready-to-heat	59	1 slice	126
French toast, prepared from recipe, made with low fat (2%) milk	65	1 slice	149
Frostings, chocolate, creamy, ready-to-eat	38	1/12 package	151
Frostings, vanilla, creamy, ready-to-eat	38	1/12 package	160
Frozen juice novelties, fruit and juice bars	77	1 bar (2.5 fl oz)	63
Frozen yogurts, chocolate, soft-serve	72	1/2 cup	115
Frozen yogurts, vanilla, soft-serve	72	1/2 cup	117
Fruit butters, apple	17	1 tbsp	29
Fruit cocktail, (peach and pineapple and pear and grape and cherry), canned, heavy syrup, solids and liquids	248	1 cup	181
Fruit cocktail, (peach and pineapple and pear and grape and cherry), canned, juice pack, solids and liquids	237	1 cup	109
Fruit punch drink, with added nutrients, canned	248	8 fl oz	117
Fruit, mixed, (peach and cherry-sweet and -sour and raspberry and grape and boysenberry), frozen, sweetened	250	1 cup	245
Garlic, raw	3	1 clove	4
Gelatin desserts, dry mix, prepared with water	135	1/2 cup	84
Gelatin desserts, dry mix, reduced calorie, with aspartame, prepared with water	117	1/2 cup	23
Grape drink, canned	250	8 fl oz	113
Grape juice, canned or bottled, unsweetened, without added vitamin C	253	1 cup	154
Grape juice, frozen concentrate, sweetened, diluted with 3 volume water, with added vitamin C	250	1 cup	128
Grape juice, frozen concentrate, sweetened, undiluted, with added vitamin C	216	6-fl-oz can	387
Grapefruit juice, pink, raw	247	1 cup	96
Grapefruit juice, white, canned, sweetened	250	1 cup	115
Grapefruit juice, white, canned, unsweetened	247	1 cup	94
Grapefruit juice, white, frozen concentrate, unsweetened, diluted with 3 volume water	247	1 cup	101
Grapefruit juice, white, frozen concentrate, unsweetened, undiluted	207	6-fl-oz can	302
Grapefruit juice, white, raw	247	1 cup	96
Grapefruit, raw, pink and red, all areas	123	1/2 grapefruit	52
Grapefruit, raw, white, all areas	118	1/2 grapefruit	39
Grapefruit, sections, canned, light syrup pack, solids and liquids	254	1 cup	152
Grapes, red or green (european type varieties, such as, Thompson seedless), raw	160	1 cup	110
Grapes, red or green (european type varieties, such as, Thompson seedless), raw	50	10 grapes	35
Gravy, beef, canned	58.25	1/4 cup	31
Gravy, chicken, canned	59.5	1/4 cup	47
Gravy, mushroom, canned	59.6	1/4 cup	30

Description	Weight (g)	Common Measure	Content per Measure
Gravy, NESTLE, CHEF-MATE Country Sausage Gravy, ready-to-serve	62	1/4 cup	96
Gravy, turkey, canned	59.6	1/4 cup	30
Ham, chopped, not canned	21	2 slices	38
Ham, sliced, extra lean	56.7	2 slices	61
Ham, sliced, regular (approximately 11% fat)	56.7	2 slices	92
HEALTHY CHOICE Beef Macaroni, frozen entree	240	1 package	211
Hearts of palm, canned	33	1 piece	9
Honey	21	1 tbsp	64
Horseradish, prepared	5	1 tsp	2
Hummus, commercial	14	1 tbsp	23
Ice creams, chocolate	66	1/2 cup	143
Ice creams, french vanilla, soft-serve	86	1/2 cup	191
Ice creams, vanilla	66	1/2 cup	133
Ice creams, vanilla, light	66	1/2 cup	109
Ice creams, vanilla, rich	74	1/2 cup	184
Ice novelties, italian, restaurant-prepared	116	1/2 cup	61
Ice novelties, pop	59	1 bar (2 fl oz)	42
Jams and preserves	20	1 tbsp	56
Jellies	19	1 tbsp	51
Jerusalem-artichokes, raw	150	1 cup	114
Kale, cooked, boiled, drained, without salt	130	1 cup	36
Kale, frozen, cooked, boiled, drained, without salt	130	1 cup	39
KELLOGG'S Eggo Lowfat Homestyle Waffles	35	1 waffle	83
Kiwi fruit, (chinese gooseberries), fresh, raw	76	1 medium	46
Kohlrabi, cooked, boiled, drained, without salt	165	1 cup	48
Lamb, domestic, leg, whole (shank and sirloin), separable lean and fat, trimmed to 1/4" fat, choice, cooked, roasted	85	3 oz	219
Lamb, domestic, leg, whole (shank and sirloin), separable lean only, trimmed to 1/4" fat, choice, cooked, roasted	85	3 oz	162
Lamb, domestic, loin, separable lean and fat, trimmed to 1/4" fat, choice, cooked, broiled	85	3 oz	269
Lamb, domestic, loin, separable lean only, trimmed to 1/4" fat, choice, cooked, broiled	85	3 oz	184
Lamb, domestic, rib, separable lean and fat, trimmed to 1/4" fat, choice, cooked, roasted	85	3 oz	305
Lamb, domestic, rib, separable lean only, trimmed to 1/4" fat, choice, cooked, roasted	85	3 oz	197
Lamb, domestic, shoulder, arm, separable lean and fat, trimmed to 1/4" fat, choice, cooked, braised	85	3 oz	294
Lamb, domestic, shoulder, arm, separable lean only, trimmed to 1/4" fat, choice, cooked, braised	85	3 oz	237
Lard	12.8	1 tbsp	115
Leavening agents, baking powder, double-acting, sodium aluminum sulfate	4.6	1 tsp	2
Leavening agents, baking powder, double-acting, straight phosphate	4.6	1 tsp	2
Leavening agents, baking powder, low-sodium	5	1 tsp	5
Leavening agents, baking soda	4.6	1 tsp	0
Leavening agents, cream of tartar	3	1 tsp	8
Leavening agents, yeast, baker's, active dry	4	1 tsp	12
Leavening agents, yeast, baker's, active dry	7	1 pkg	21
Leavening agents, yeast, baker's, compressed	17	1 cake	18

Description	Weight (g)	Common Measure	Content per Measure
Leeks, (bulb and lower leaf-portion), cooked, boiled, drained, without salt	104	1 cup	32
Lemon juice, canned or bottled	15.2	1 tbsp	3
Lemon juice, canned or bottled	244	1 cup	51
Lemon juice, raw	47	juice of 1 lemon	12
Lemonade, frozen concentrate, white, prepared with water	248	8 fl oz	131
Lemonade, low calorie, with aspartame, powder, prepared with water	237	8 fl oz	5
Lemonade-flavor drink, powder, prepared with water	266	8 fl oz	112
Lemons, raw, without peel	58	1 lemon	17
Lentils, mature seeds, cooked, boiled, without salt	198	1 cup	230
Lettuce, butterhead (includes boston and bibb types), raw	7.5	1 medium leaf	1
Lettuce, butterhead (includes boston and bibb types), raw	163	1 head	21
Lettuce, cos or romaine, raw	10	1 leaf	2
Lettuce, cos or romaine, raw	56	1 cup	10
Lettuce, green leaf, raw	10	1 leaf	2
Lettuce, green leaf, raw	56	1 cup	8
Lettuce, iceberg (includes crisphead types), raw	8	1 medium	1
Lettuce, iceberg (includes crisphead types), raw	539	1 head	75
Lettuce, iceberg (includes crisphead types), raw	55	1 cup	8
Lima beans, immature seeds, frozen, baby, cooked, boiled, drained, without salt	180	1 cup	189
Lima beans, immature seeds, frozen, fordhook, cooked, boiled, drained, without salt	170	1 cup	175
Lima beans, large, mature seeds, canned	241	1 cup	190
Lima beans, large, mature seeds, cooked, boiled, without salt	188	1 cup	216
Lime juice, canned or bottled, unsweetened	15.4	1 tbsp	3
Lime juice, canned or bottled, unsweetened	246	1 cup	52
Lime juice, raw	38	juice of 1 lime	10
Macaroni and Cheese, canned entree	252	1 cup	207
Macaroni, cooked, enriched	140	1 cup	197
Malted drink mix, chocolate, with added nutrients, powder	21	3 heaping tsp	79
Malted drink mix, chocolate, with added nutrients, powder, prepared with whole milk	265	1 cup	223
Malted drink mix, natural, with added nutrients, powder	21	4-5 heaping tsp	80
Malted drink mix, natural, with added nutrients, powder, prepared with whole milk	265	1 cup	228
Mangos, raw	165	1 cup	107
Mangos, raw	207	1 mango	135
Margarine, regular, tub, composite, 80% fat, with salt	14.2	1 tbsp	102
Margarine, regular, unspecified oils, with salt added	14.1	1 tbsp	101
Margarine, vegetable oil spread, 60% fat, stick	14.3	1 tbsp	74
Margarine, vegetable oil spread, 60% fat, stick	4.8	1 tsp	25
Margarine, vegetable oil spread, 60% fat, tub/bottle	4.8	1 tsp	25
Margarine-butter blend, 60% corn oil margarine and 40% butter	14.2	1 tbsp	102
Margarine-like spread, (approximately 40% fat), unspecified oils	4.8	1 tsp	17
Melons, cantaloupe, raw	69	1/8 melon	23
Melons, cantaloupe, raw	160	1 cup	54
Melons, honeydew, raw	170	1 cup	61
Melons, honeydew, raw	160	1/8 melon	58
Milk shakes, thick chocolate	300	10.6 fl oz	357

Description	Weight (g)	Common Measure	Content per Measure
Milk shakes, thick vanilla	313	11 fl oz	351
Milk, buttermilk, dried	6.5	1 tbsp	25
Milk, buttermilk, fluid, cultured, lowfat	245	1 cup	98
Milk, canned, condensed, sweetened	306	1 cup	982
Milk, canned, evaporated, nonfat	256	1 cup	200
Milk, canned, evaporated, without added vitamin A	252	1 cup	338
Milk, chocolate, fluid, commercial,	250	1 cup	208
Milk, chocolate, fluid, commercial, lowfat	250	1 cup	158
Milk, chocolate, fluid, commercial, reduced fat	250	1 cup	180
Milk, dry, nonfat, instant, with added vitamin A	23	1/3 cup	82
Milk, lowfat, fluid, 1% milkfat, with added vitamin A	244	1 cup	102
Milk, nonfat, fluid, with added vitamin A (fat free or skim)	245	1 cup	83
Milk, reduced fat, fluid, 2% milkfat, with added vitamin A	244	1 cup	122
Milk, whole, 3.25% milkfat	244	1 cup	146
Miso	68.75	1 cup	137
Molasses, blackstrap	20	1 tbsp	47
Mollusks, clam, mixed species, canned, drained solids	85	3 oz	126
Mollusks, clam, mixed species, raw	85	3 oz	63
Mollusks, oyster, eastern, cooked, breaded and fried	85	3 oz	167
Mollusks, oyster, eastern, wild, raw	84	6 medium	57
Mollusks, scallop, mixed species, cooked, breaded and fried	93	6 large	200
Muffins, blueberry, commercially prepared	57	1 muffin	158
Muffins, blueberry, prepared from recipe, made with low fat (2%) milk	57	1 muffin	162
Muffins, corn, commercially prepared	57	1 muffin	174
Muffins, corn, dry mix, prepared	50	1 muffin	161
Muffins, oat bran	57	1 muffin	154
Muffins, wheat bran, toaster-type with raisins, toasted	34	1 muffin	106
Mung beans, mature seeds, sprouted, cooked, boiled, drained, without salt	124	1 cup	26
Mung beans, mature seeds, sprouted, raw	104	1 cup	31
Mushrooms, canned, drained solids	156	1 cup	39
Mushrooms, cooked, boiled, drained, without salt	156	1 cup	44
Mushrooms, raw	70	1 cup	15
Mushrooms, shiitake, cooked, without salt	145	1 cup	80
Mushrooms, shiitake, dried	3.6	1 mushroom	11
Mustard greens, cooked, boiled, drained, without salt	140	1 cup	21
Mustard, prepared, yellow	5	1 tsp or 1 packet	3
NABISCO, NABISCO SNACKWELL'S Fat Free Devil's Food Cookie Cakes	16	1 cookie	49
Nectarines, raw	136	1 nectarine	60
Noodles, chinese, chow mein	45	1 cup	237
Noodles, egg, cooked, enriched	160	1 cup	213
Noodles, egg, spinach, cooked, enriched	160	1 cup	211
Nuts, almonds	28.35	1 oz (24 nuts)	164
Nuts, brazilnuts, dried, unblanched	28.35	1 oz (6-8 nuts)	186
Nuts, cashew nuts, dry roasted, with salt added	28.35	1 oz	163
Nuts, cashew nuts, oil roasted, with salt added	28.35	1 oz (18 nuts)	165
Nuts, chestnuts, european, roasted	143	1 cup	350
Nuts, coconut meat, dried (desiccated), sweetened, shredded	93	1 cup	466

Description	Weight (g)	Common Measure	Content per Measure
Nuts, coconut meat, raw	45	1 piece	159
Nuts, hazelnuts or filberts	28.35	1 oz	178
Nuts, macadamia nuts, dry roasted, with salt added	28.35	1 oz (10-12 nuts)	203
Nuts, mixed nuts, dry roasted, with peanuts, with salt added	28.35	1 oz	168
Nuts, mixed nuts, oil roasted, with peanuts, with salt added	28.35	1 oz	175
Nuts, pecans	28.35	1 oz (20 halves)	196
Nuts, pine nuts, dried	8.6	1 tbsp	58
Nuts, pine nuts, dried	28.35	1 oz	191
Nuts, pistachio nuts, dry roasted, with salt added	28.35	1 oz (47 nuts)	161
Nuts, walnuts, english	28.35	1 oz (14 halves)	185
Oat bran, cooked	219	1 cup	88
Oat bran, raw	94	1 cup	231
Oil, olive, salad or cooking	13.5	1 tbsp	119
Oil, peanut, salad or cooking	13.5	1 tbsp	119
Oil, sesame, salad or cooking	13.6	1 tbsp	120
Oil, soybean, salad or cooking, (hydrogenated)	13.6	1 tbsp	120
Oil, soybean, salad or cooking, (hydrogenated) and cottonseed	13.6	1 tbsp	120
Oil, vegetable safflower, salad or cooking, oleic, over 70% (primary safflower oil of commerce)	13.6	1 tbsp	120
Oil, vegetable, corn, industrial and retail, all purpose salad or cooking	13.6	1 tbsp	120
Oil, vegetable, sunflower, linoleic, (approx. 65%)	13.6	1 tbsp	120
Okra, cooked, boiled, drained, without salt	160	1 cup	35
Okra, frozen, cooked, boiled, drained, without salt	184	1 cup	52
Olives, ripe, canned (small-extra large)	22	5 large	25
Onion rings, breaded, par fried, frozen, prepared, heated in oven	60	10 rings	244
Onions, cooked, boiled, drained, without salt	210	1 cup	92
Onions, cooked, boiled, drained, without salt	94	1 medium	41
Onions, dehydrated flakes	5	1 tbsp	17
Onions, raw	110	1 whole	46
Onions, raw	14	1 slice	6
Onions, raw	160	1 cup	67
Onions, spring or scallions (includes tops and bulb), raw	100	1 cup	32
Onions, spring or scallions (includes tops and bulb), raw	15	1 whole	5
Orange juice, canned, unsweetened	249	1 cup	105
Orange juice, chilled, includes from concentrate	249	1 cup	110
Orange juice, frozen concentrate, unsweetened, diluted with 3 volume water	249	1 cup	112
Orange juice, frozen concentrate, unsweetened, undiluted	213	6-fl-oz can	339
Orange juice, raw	86	juice from 1 orange	39
Orange juice, raw	248	1 cup	112
Oranges, raw, all commercial varieties	180	1 cup	85
Oranges, raw, all commercial varieties	131	1 orange	62
Pancakes plain, frozen, ready-to-heat (includes buttermilk)	36	1 pancake	82
Pancakes, plain, dry mix, complete, prepared	38	1 pancake	74
Pancakes, plain, dry mix, incomplete, prepared	38	1 pancake	83
Papayas, raw	140	1 cup	55
Papayas, raw	304	1 papaya	119
Parsley, raw	10	10 sprigs	4
Parsnips, cooked, boiled, drained, without salt	156	1 cup	111

Description	Weight (g)	Common Measure	Content per Measure
Pasta with meatballs in tomato sauce, canned entree	252	1 cup	260
Peaches, canned, heavy syrup pack, solids and liquids	262	1 cup	194
Peaches, canned, heavy syrup pack, solids and liquids	98	1 half	73
Peaches, canned, juice pack, solids and liquids	98	1 half	43
Peaches, canned, juice pack, solids and liquids	248	1 cup	109
Peaches, dried, sulfured, uncooked	39	3 halves	93
Peaches, frozen, sliced, sweetened	250	1 cup	235
Peaches, raw	170	1 cup	66
Peaches, raw	98	1 peach	38
Peanut butter, chunk style, with salt	16	1 tbsp	94
Peanut butter, smooth style, with salt	16	1 tbsp	94
Peanuts, all types, dry-roasted, with salt	28.35	1 oz (approx 28)	166
Peanuts, all types, dry-roasted, without salt	28.35	1 oz (approx 28)	166
Peanuts, all types, oil-roasted, with salt	28.35	1 oz	170
Pears, asian, raw	122	1 pear	51
Pears, asian, raw	275	1 pear	116
Pears, canned, heavy syrup pack, solids and liquids	266	1 cup	197
Pears, canned, heavy syrup pack, solids and liquids	76	1 half	56
Pears, canned, juice pack, solids and liquids	248	1 cup	124
Pears, canned, juice pack, solids and liquids	76	1 half	38
Pears, raw	166	1 pear	96
Peas, edible-podded, cooked, boiled, drained, without salt	160	1 cup	67
Peas, edible-podded, frozen, cooked, boiled, drained, without salt	160	1 cup	83
Peas, green, canned, regular pack, drained solids	170	1 cup	117
Peas, green, frozen, cooked, boiled, drained, without salt	160	1 cup	125
Peas, split, mature seeds, cooked, boiled, without salt	196	1 cup	231
Peppers, hot chili, green, raw	45	1 pepper	18
Peppers, hot chili, red, raw	45	1 pepper	18
Peppers, jalapeno, canned, solids and liquids	26	1/4 cup	7
Peppers, sweet, green, cooked, boiled, drained, without salt	136	1 cup	38
Peppers, sweet, green, raw	149	1 cup	30
Peppers, sweet, green, raw	10	1 ring	2
Peppers, sweet, green, raw	119	1 pepper	24
Peppers, sweet, red, cooked, boiled, drained, without salt	136	1 cup	38
Peppers, sweet, red, raw	119	1 pepper	31
Peppers, sweet, red, raw	149	1 cup	39
Pickle relish, sweet	15	1 tbsp	20
Pickles, cucumber, dill	65	1 pickle	12
Pie crust, cookie-type, prepared from recipe, graham cracker, baked	239	1 pie shell	1181
Pie crust, standard-type, frozen, ready-to-bake, baked	126	1 pie shell	648
Pie crust, standard-type, prepared from recipe, baked	180	1 pie shell	949
Pie fillings, apple, canned	74	1/8 of 21-oz can	75
Pie fillings, canned, cherry	74	1/8 of 21-oz can	85
Pie, apple, commercially prepared, enriched flour	117	1 piece	277
Pie, apple, prepared from recipe	155	1 piece	411
Pie, blueberry, commercially prepared	117	1 piece	271
Pie, blueberry, prepared from recipe	147	1 piece	360
Pie, cherry, commercially prepared	117	1 piece	304

Description	Weight (g)	Common Measure	Content per Measure
Pie, cherry, prepared from recipe	180	1 piece	486
Pie, chocolate creme, commercially prepared	113	1 piece	344
Pie, coconut custard, commercially prepared	104	1 piece	270
Pie, fried pies, cherry	128	1 pie	404
Pie, fried pies, fruit	128	1 pie	404
Pie, lemon meringue, commercially prepared	113	1 piece	303
Pie, lemon meringue, prepared from recipe	127	1 piece	362
Pie, pecan, commercially prepared	113	1 piece	452
Pie, pecan, prepared from recipe	122	1 piece	503
Pie, pumpkin, commercially prepared	109	1 piece	229
Pie, pumpkin, prepared from recipe	155	1 piece	316
Pimento, canned	12	1 tbsp	3
Pineapple and grapefruit juice drink, canned	250	8 fl oz	118
Pineapple and orange juice drink, canned	250	8 fl oz	125
Pineapple juice, canned, unsweetened, without added ascorbic acid	250	1 cup	140
Pineapple, canned, heavy syrup pack, solids and liquids	49	1 slice	38
Pineapple, canned, heavy syrup pack, solids and liquids	254	1 cup	198
Pineapple, canned, juice pack, solids and liquids	47	1 slice	28
Pineapple, canned, juice pack, solids and liquids	249	1 cup	149
Pineapple, raw, all varieties	155	1 cup	74
Pizza, cheese, regular crust, frozen	63	1 serving	169
Pizza, meat and vegetable, regular crust, frozen	79	1 serving	218
Plantains, cooked	154	1 cup	179
Plantains, raw	179	1 medium	218
Plums, canned, purple, heavy syrup pack, solids and liquids	258	1 cup	230
Plums, canned, purple, heavy syrup pack, solids and liquids	46	1 plum	41
Plums, canned, purple, juice pack, solids and liquids	46	1 plum	27
Plums, canned, purple, juice pack, solids and liquids	252	1 cup	146
Plums, dried (prunes), stewed, without added sugar	248	1 cup	265
Plums, dried (prunes), uncooked	42	5 prunes	101
Plums, raw	66	1 plum	30
Pork and beef sausage, fresh, cooked	26	2 links	103
Pork sausage, fresh, cooked	26	2 links	88
Pork sausage, fresh, cooked	27	1 patty	92
Pork, cured, bacon, cooked, broiled, pan-fried or roasted	19	3 medium slices	103
Pork, cured, canadian-style bacon, grilled	46.5	2 slices	86
Pork, cured, ham, extra lean and regular, canned, roasted	85	3 oz	142
Pork, cured, ham, whole, separable lean and fat, roasted	85	3 oz	207
Pork, cured, ham, whole, separable lean only, roasted	85	3 oz	133
Pork, fresh, backribs, separable lean and fat, cooked, roasted	85	3 oz	315
Pork, fresh, leg (ham), whole, separable lean and fat, cooked, roasted	85	3 oz	232
Pork, fresh, leg (ham), whole, separable lean only, cooked, roasted	85	3 oz	179
Pork, fresh, loin, center loin (chops), bone-in, separable lean and fat, cooked, broiled	85	3 oz	204
Pork, fresh, loin, center loin (chops), bone-in, separable lean and fat, cooked, pan-fried	85	3 oz	235
Pork, fresh, loin, center loin (chops), bone-in, separable lean only, cooked, broiled	85	3 oz	172
Pork, fresh, loin, center loin (chops), bone-in, separable lean only, cooked, pan-fried	85	3 oz	197

Description	Weight (g)	Common Measure	Content per Measure
Pork, fresh, loin, center rib (roasts), bone-in, separable lean and fat, cooked, roasted	85	3 oz	217
Pork, fresh, loin, center rib (roasts), bone-in, separable lean only, cooked, roasted	85	3 oz	190
Pork, fresh, loin, country-style ribs, separable lean and fat, cooked, braised	85	3 oz	252
Pork, fresh, shoulder, arm picnic, separable lean and fat, cooked, braised	85	3 oz	280
Pork, fresh, shoulder, arm picnic, separable lean only, cooked, braised	85	3 oz	211
Pork, fresh, spareribs, separable lean and fat, cooked, braised	85	3 oz	337
Potato pancakes, home-prepared	76	1 pancake	207
Potato puffs, frozen, prepared	79	10 puffs	175
Potato salad, home-prepared	250	1 cup	358
Potato, baked, flesh and skin, without salt	202	1 potato	188
Potatoes, au gratin, dry mix, prepared with water, whole milk and butter	245	1 cup	228
Potatoes, au gratin, home-prepared from recipe using butter	245	1 cup	323
Potatoes, baked, flesh, without salt	156	1 potato	145
Potatoes, baked, skin, without salt	58	1 skin	115
Potatoes, boiled, cooked in skin, flesh, without salt	136	1 potato	118
Potatoes, boiled, cooked without skin, flesh, without salt	156	1 cup	134
Potatoes, boiled, cooked without skin, flesh, without salt	135	1 potato	116
Potatoes, french fried, frozen, home-prepared, heated in oven, without salt	50	10 strips	100
Potatoes, hashed brown, frozen, plain, prepared	29	1 patty	63
Potatoes, hashed brown, home-prepared	156	1 cup	413
Potatoes, mashed, dehydrated, prepared from flakes without milk, whole milk and butter added	210	1 cup	204
Potatoes, mashed, home-prepared, whole milk added	210	1 cup	174
Potatoes, mashed, home-prepared, whole milk and margarine added	210	1 cup	237
Potatoes, scalloped, dry mix, prepared with water, whole milk and butter	245	1 cup	228
Potatoes, scalloped, home-prepared with butter	245	1 cup	211
Poultry food products, ground turkey, cooked	82	1 patty	193
Prune juice, canned	256	1 cup	182
Puddings, chocolate, dry mix, instant, prepared with 2% milk	147	1/2 cup	154
Puddings, chocolate, dry mix, regular, prepared with 2% milk	142	1/2 cup	155
Puddings, chocolate, ready-to-eat	113	4 oz	157
Puddings, rice, ready-to-eat	113.4	4 oz	185
Puddings, tapioca, ready-to-eat	113	4 oz	134
Puddings, vanilla, dry mix, regular, prepared with 2% milk	140	1/2 cup	141
Puddings, vanilla, ready-to-eat	113	4 oz	146
Pumpkin, canned, without salt	245	1 cup	83
Pumpkin, cooked, boiled, drained, without salt	245	1 cup	49
Radishes, raw	4.5	1 radish	1
Raisins, seedless	14	1 packet	42
Raisins, seedless	145	1 cup	434
Raspberries, frozen, red, sweetened	250	1 cup	258
Raspberries, raw	123	1 cup	64
Refried beans, canned (includes USDA commodity)	252	1 cup	237
Rhubarb, frozen, cooked, with sugar	240	1 cup	278
Rice beverage, RICE DREAM, canned	245	1 cup	120

Description	Weight (g)	Common Measure	Content per Measure
Rice, brown, long-grain, cooked	195	1 cup	216
Rice, white, long-grain, parboiled, enriched, cooked	175	1 cup	200
Rice, white, long-grain, parboiled, enriched, dry	185	1 cup	686
Rice, white, long-grain, precooked or instant, enriched, prepared	165	1 cup	162
Rice, white, long-grain, regular, cooked	158	1 cup	205
Rice, white, long-grain, regular, raw, enriched	185	1 cup	675
Rolls, dinner, plain, commercially prepared (includes brown-and-serve)	28	1 roll	84
Rolls, hamburger or hotdog, plain	43	1 roll	120
Rolls, hard (includes kaiser)	57	1 roll	167
Rutabagas, cooked, boiled, drained, without salt	170	1 cup	66
Salad dressing, blue or roquefort cheese dressing, commercial, regular	15.3	1 tbsp	77
Salad dressing, french dressing, commercial, regular	15.6	1 tbsp	71
Salad dressing, french dressing, reduced fat	16.3	1 tbsp	38
Salad dressing, french, home recipe	14	1 tbsp	88
Salad dressing, home recipe, cooked	16	1 tbsp	25
Salad dressing, home recipe, vinegar and oil	15.6	1 tbsp	70
Salad dressing, italian dressing, commercial, regular	14.7	1 tbsp	43
Salad dressing, italian dressing, reduced fat	15	1 tbsp	11
Salad dressing, mayonnaise, soybean oil, with salt	13.8	1 tbsp	99
Salad dressing, russian dressing	15.3	1 tbsp	76
Salad dressing, russian dressing, low calorie	16.3	1 tbsp	23
Salad dressing, thousand island dressing, reduced fat	15.3	1 tbsp	31
Salad dressing, thousand island, commercial, regular	15.6	1 tbsp	58
Salami, cooked, beef and pork	56.7	2 slices	142
Salami, dry or hard, pork, beef	20	2 slices	77
Salt, table	6	1 tsp	0
Sandwich spread, pork, beef	15	1 tbsp	35
Sandwiches and burgers, cheeseburger, large, single meat patty, with bacon and condiments	195	1 sandwich	608
Sandwiches and burgers, cheeseburger, regular, single meat patty, plain	102	1 sandwich	319
Sandwiches and burgers, hamburger, large, single meat patty, with condiments and vegetables	218	1 sandwich	512
Sauce, barbecue sauce	15.75	1 tbsp	12
Sauce, cheese, ready-to-serve	63	1/4 cup	110
Sauce, hoisin, ready-to-serve	16	1 tbsp	35
Sauce, homemade, white, medium	250	1 cup	368
Sauce, NESTLE, ORTEGA Mild Nacho Cheese Sauce, ready-to-serve	63	1/4 cup	119
Sauce, pasta, spaghetti/marinara, ready-to-serve	250	1 cup	185
Sauce, ready-to-serve, pepper or hot	4.7	1 tsp	1
Sauce, ready-to-serve, salsa	16	1 tbsp	4
Sauce, teriyaki, ready-to-serve	18	1 tbsp	15
Sauerkraut, canned, solids and liquids	236	1 cup	45
Sausage, Vienna, canned, chicken, beef, pork	16	1 sausage	37
Seaweed, kelp, raw	10	2 tbsp	4
Seaweed, spirulina, dried	0.93	1 tbsp	3
Seeds, pumpkin and squash seed kernels, roasted, with salt added	28.35	1 oz (142 seeds)	148
Seeds, sesame butter, tahini, from roasted and toasted kernels (most common type)	15	1 tbsp	89

Description	Weight (g)	Common Measure	Content per Measure
Seeds, sesame seed kernels, dried (decorticated)	8	1 tbsp	47
Seeds, sunflower seed kernels, dry roasted, with salt added	28.35	1 oz	165
Seeds, sunflower seed kernels, dry roasted, with salt added	32	1/4 cup	186
Shake, fast food, chocolate	333	16 fl oz	423
Shake, fast food, vanilla	333	16 fl oz	370
Shallots, raw	10	1 tbsp	7
Sherbet, orange	74	1/2 cup	107
Shortening, household, soybean (hydrogenated)-cottonseed (hydrogenated)	12.8	1 tbsp	113
Snacks, beef jerky, chopped and formed	19.8	1 large piece	81
Snacks, CHEX mix	28.35	1 oz (about 2/3 cup)	120
Snacks, corn-based, extruded, chips, barbecue-flavor	28.35	1 oz	148
Snacks, corn-based, extruded, chips, plain	28.35	1 oz	153
Snacks, corn-based, extruded, puffs or twists, cheese-flavor	28.35	1 oz	157
Snacks, fruit leather, pieces	28.35	1 oz	100
Snacks, fruit leather, rolls	21	1 large	78
Snacks, granola bars, hard, plain	28.35	1 bar	134
Snacks, granola bars, soft, coated, milk chocolate coating, peanut butter	28.35	1 bar	144
Snacks, granola bars, soft, uncoated, chocolate chip	28.35	1 bar	119
Snacks, granola bars, soft, uncoated, raisin	28.35	1 bar	127
Snacks, KELLOGG, KELLOGGS NUTRI-GRAIN Cereal Bars, fruit	37	1 bar	136
Snacks, KELLOGG, KELLOGGS RICE KRISPIES TREATS Squares	22	1 bar	91
Snacks, oriental mix, rice-based	28.35	1 oz (about 1/4 cup)	143
Snacks, popcorn, air-popped	8	1 cup	31
Snacks, popcorn, cakes	10	1 cake	38
Snacks, popcorn, caramel-coated, with peanuts	42	1 cup	168
Snacks, popcorn, caramel-coated, without peanuts	35.2	1 cup	152
Snacks, popcorn, cheese-flavor	11	1 cup	58
Snacks, popcorn, oil-popped	11	1 cup	55
Snacks, pork skins, plain	28.35	1 oz	155
Snacks, potato chips, barbecue-flavor	28.35	1 oz	139
Snacks, potato chips, made from dried potatoes, light	28.35	1 oz	142
Snacks, potato chips, made from dried potatoes, plain	28.35	1 oz	158
Snacks, potato chips, made from dried potatoes, sour-cream and onion-flavor	28.35	1 oz	155
Snacks, potato chips, plain, salted	28.35	1 oz	152
Snacks, potato chips, plain, unsalted	28.35	1 oz	152
Snacks, potato chips, reduced fat	28.35	1 oz	134
Snacks, potato chips, sour-cream-and-onion-flavor	28.35	1 oz	151
Snacks, pretzels, hard, plain, salted	60	10 pretzels	229
Snacks, rice cakes, brown rice, plain	9	1 cake	35
Snacks, tortilla chips, nacho-flavor	28.35	1 oz	141
Snacks, tortilla chips, nacho-flavor, reduced fat	28.35	1 oz	126
Snacks, tortilla chips, plain	28.35	1 oz	142
Snacks, trail mix, regular, with chocolate chips, salted nuts and seeds	146	1 cup	707
Snacks, trail mix, tropical	140	1 cup	570
Soup, bean with ham, canned, chunky, ready-to-serve, commercial	243	1 cup	231
Soup, bean with pork, canned, prepared with equal volume water, commercial	253	1 cup	172

Description	Weight (g)	Common Measure	Content per Measure
Soup, beef broth or bouillon, powder, dry	6	1 packet	14
Soup, beef broth, bouillon, consomme, prepared with equal volume water, commercial	241	1 cup	29
Soup, beef noodle, canned, prepared with equal volume water, commercial	244	1 cup	83
Soup, chicken noodle, canned, chunky, ready-to-serve	240	1 cup	175
Soup, chicken noodle, canned, prepared with equal volume water, commercial	241	1 cup	75
Soup, chicken noodle, dehydrated, prepared with water	252.3	1 cup	58
Soup, chicken vegetable, canned, chunky, ready-to-serve	240	1 cup	166
Soup, chicken with rice, canned, prepared with equal volume water, commercial	241	1 cup	60
Soup, clam chowder, manhattan, canned, prepared with equal volume water	244	1 cup	78
Soup, clam chowder, new england, canned, prepared with equal volume milk, commercial	248	1 cup	164
Soup, cream of chicken, canned, prepared with equal volume water, commercial	244	1 cup	117
Soup, cream of chicken, prepared with equal volume milk, commercial	248	1 cup	191
Soup, cream of mushroom, canned, prepared with equal volume milk, commercial	248	1 cup	203
Soup, cream of mushroom, canned, prepared with equal volume water, commercial	244	1 cup	129
Soup, minestrone, canned, prepared with equal volume water, commercial	241	1 cup	82
Soup, onion mix, dehydrated, dry form	39	1 packet	118
Soup, onion, dehydrated, prepared with water	246	1 cup	27
Soup, pea, green, canned, prepared with equal volume water, commercial	250	1 cup	165
Soup, PROGRESSO HEALTHY CLASSICS CHICKEN NOODLE, canned, ready-to-serve	237	1 cup	76
Soup, PROGRESSO HEALTHY CLASSICS CHICKEN RICE WITH VEGETABLES, canned, ready-to-serve	239	1 cup	88
Soup, PROGRESSO HEALTHY CLASSICS LENTIL, canned, ready-to-serve	242	1 cup	126
Soup, PROGRESSO HEALTHY CLASSICS MINESTRONE, canned, ready-to-serve	241	1 cup	123
Soup, PROGRESSO HEALTHY CLASSICS NEW ENGLAND CLAM CHOWDER, canned, ready-to-serve	244	1 cup	117
Soup, PROGRESSO HEALTHY CLASSICS VEGETABLE, canned, ready-to-serve	238	1 cup	81
Soup, stock, fish, home-prepared	233	1 cup	40
Soup, tomato, canned, prepared with equal volume milk, commercial	248	1 cup	161
Soup, tomato, canned, prepared with equal volume water, commercial	244	1 cup	85
Soup, vegetable beef, prepared with equal volume water, commercial	244	1 cup	78
Soup, vegetable, canned, chunky, ready-to-serve, commercial	240	1 cup	122
Soup, vegetarian vegetable, canned, prepared with equal volume water, commercial	241	1 cup	72
Sour dressing, non-butterfat, cultured, filled cream-type	12	1 tbsp	21
Soy milk, fluid	245	1 cup	127
Soy sauce made from soy and wheat (shoyu)	16	1 tbsp	8
Soybeans, green, cooked, boiled, drained, without salt	180	1 cup	254
Soybeans, mature cooked, boiled, without salt	172	1 cup	298
Spaghetti with meat sauce, frozen entree	283	1 package	255
Spaghetti, cooked, enriched, without added salt	140	1 cup	197
Spaghetti, whole-wheat, cooked	140	1 cup	174

Description	Weight (g)	Common Measure	Content per Measure
Spices, celery seed	2	1 tsp	8
Spices, chili powder	2.6	1 tsp	8
Spices, cinnamon, ground	2.3	1 tsp	6
Spices, curry powder	2	1 tsp	7
Spices, garlic powder	2.8	1 tsp	9
Spices, onion powder	2.1	1 tsp	7
Spices, oregano, dried	1.5	1 tsp	5
Spices, paprika	2.1	1 tsp	6
Spices, parsley, dried	1.3	1 tbsp	4
Spices, pepper, black	2.1	1 tsp	5
Spinach souffle, home-prepared	136	1 cup	219
Spinach, canned, drained solids	214	1 cup	49
Spinach, cooked, boiled, drained, without salt	180	1 cup	41
Spinach, frozen, chopped or leaf, cooked, boiled, drained, without salt	190	1 cup	61
Spinach, raw	30	1 cup	7
Spinach, raw	10	1 leaf	2
Squash, summer, all varieties, cooked, boiled, drained, without salt	180	1 cup	36
Squash, summer, all varieties, raw	113	1 cup	18
Squash, winter, all varieties, cooked, baked, without salt	205	1 cup	76
Squash, winter, butternut, frozen, cooked, boiled, without salt	240	1 cup	94
Strawberries, frozen, sweetened, sliced	255	1 cup	245
Strawberries, raw	166	1 cup	53
Strawberries, raw	18	1 strawberry	6
Strawberries, raw	12	1 strawberry	4
Sugars, brown	3.2	1 tsp	12
Sugars, granulated	4.2	1 tsp	16
Sugars, powdered	8	1 tbsp	31
Sweet potato, canned, syrup pack, drained solids	196	1 cup	212
Sweet potato, canned, vacuum pack	255	1 cup	232
Sweet potato, cooked, baked in skin, without salt	146	1 potato	131
Sweet potato, cooked, boiled, without skin	156	1 potato	119
Sweet potato, cooked, candied, home-prepared	105	1 piece	151
Sweet rolls, cinnamon, commercially prepared with raisins	60	1 roll	223
Sweet rolls, cinnamon, refrigerated dough with frosting, baked	30	1 roll	109
Syrups, chocolate, fudge-type	19	1 tbsp	67
Syrups, corn, light	20	1 tbsp	59
Syrups, maple	20	1 tbsp	52
Syrups, table blends, pancake	20	1 tbsp	47
Syrups, table blends, pancake, reduced-calorie	15	1 tbsp	25
Taco shells, baked	13.3	1 medium	62
Tangerine juice, canned, sweetened	249	1 cup	125
Tangerines, (mandarin oranges), canned, light syrup pack	252	1 cup	154
Tangerines, (mandarin oranges), raw	84	1 tangerine	45
Tapioca, pearl, dry	152	1 cup	544
Tea, brewed, prepared with tap water	178	6 fl oz	2
Tea, herb, chamomile, brewed	178	6 fl oz	2
Tea, herb, other than chamomile, brewed	178	6 fl oz	2
Tea, instant, sweetened with sodium saccharin, lemon-flavored, prepared	237	8 fl oz	5

Description	Weight (g)	Common Measure	Content per Measure
Tea, instant, sweetened with sugar, lemon-flavored, without added ascorbic acid, powder, prepared	259	8 fl oz	88
Tea, instant, unsweetened, powder, prepared	237	8 fl oz	2
Toaster pastries, brown-sugar-cinnamon	50	1 pastry	206
Toaster pastries, fruit (includes apple, blueberry, cherry, strawberry)	52	1 pastry	204
Toaster Pastries, KELLOGG, KELLOGG'S POP TARTS, Frosted chocolate fudge	52	1 pastry	201
Tofu, firm, prepared with calcium sulfate and magnesium chloride (nigari)	81	1/4 block	57
Tofu, soft, prepared with calcium sulfate and magnesium chloride (nigari)	120	1 piece	73
Tomatillos, raw	34	1 medium	11
Tomato juice, canned, with salt added	243	1 cup	41
Tomato products, canned, paste, without salt added	262	1 cup	215
Tomato products, canned, puree, without salt added	250	1 cup	95
Tomato products, canned, sauce	245	1 cup	78
Tomatoes, red, ripe, canned, stewed	255	1 cup	66
Tomatoes, red, ripe, canned, whole, regular pack	240	1 cup	41
Tomatoes, red, ripe, raw, year round average	180	1 cup	32
Tomatoes, red, ripe, raw, year round average	17	1 cherry tomato	3
Tomatoes, red, ripe, raw, year round average	20	1 slice	4
Tomatoes, red, ripe, raw, year round average	123	1 tomato	22
Tomatoes, sun-dried	2	1 piece	5
Tomatoes, sun-dried, packed in oil, drained	3	1 piece	6
Tortillas, ready-to-bake or -fry, corn	26	1 tortilla	57
Tortillas, ready-to-bake or -fry, flour	32	1 tortilla	100
Tostada with guacamole	130.5	1 tostada	180
Turkey and gravy, frozen	142	5-oz package	95
Turkey patties, breaded, battered, fried	64	1 patty	181
Turkey roast, boneless, frozen, seasoned, light and dark meat, roasted	85.05	3 oz	132
Turkey, all classes, dark meat, cooked, roasted	84	3 oz	157
Turkey, all classes, giblets, cooked, simmered, some giblet fat	145	1 cup	289
Turkey, all classes, light meat, cooked, roasted	84	3 oz	132
Turkey, all classes, meat only, cooked, roasted	140	1 cup	238
Turkey, all classes, neck, meat only, cooked, simmered	152	1 neck	274
Turnip greens, cooked, boiled, drained, without salt	144	1 cup	29
Turnip greens, frozen, cooked, boiled, drained, without salt	164	1 cup	48
Turnips, cooked, boiled, drained, without salt	156	1 cup	34
Vanilla extract	4.2	1 tsp	12
Veal, leg (top round), separable lean and fat, cooked, braised	85	3 oz	179
Veal, rib, separable lean and fat, cooked, roasted	85	3 oz	194
Vegetable juice cocktail, canned	242	1 cup	46
Vegetable oil, canola	14	1 tbsp	124
Vegetables, mixed, canned, drained solids	163	1 cup	80
Vegetables, mixed, frozen, cooked, boiled, drained, without salt	182	1 cup	118
Vinegar, cider	15	1 tbsp	2
Waffles, plain, frozen, ready-to-heat, toasted (includes buttermilk)	33	1 waffle	87
Waffles, plain, prepared from recipe	75	1 waffle	218
Water, municipal	237	8 fl oz	0
Waterchestnuts, chinese, canned, solids and liquids	140	1 cup	70

Description	Weight (g)	Common Measure	Content per Measure
Watermelon, raw	286	1 wedge	86
Watermelon, raw	152	1 cup	46
Wheat flour, white, all-purpose, enriched, bleached	125	1 cup	455
Wheat flour, white, all-purpose, self-rising, enriched	125	1 cup	443
Wheat flour, white, bread, enriched	137	1 cup	495
Wheat flour, white, cake, enriched	137	1 cup	496
Wheat flour, whole-grain	120	1 cup	407
Wild rice, cooked	164	1 cup	166
WORTHINGTON FOODS, MORNINGSTAR FARMS "Burger" Crumbles	110	1 cup	231
WORTHINGTON FOODS, MORNINGSTAR FARMS BETTERN BURGERS, frozen	85	1 patty	91
Yogurt, fruit, low fat, 10 grams protein per 8 ounce	227	8-oz container	232
Yogurt, plain, low fat, 12 grams protein per 8 ounce	227	8-oz container	143
Yogurt, plain, skim milk, 13 grams protein per 8 ounce	227	8-oz container	127
Yogurt, plain, whole milk, 8 grams protein per 8 ounce	227	8-oz container	138

Appendix III: *Table of Calories by Activity*

Activity Per Hour	Calories Burned by Weight in Pounds					
	130	155	190	210	250	300
Running, 10 mph (6 min mile)	944	1126	1380	1525	1816	2179
Running, 10.9 mph (5.5 min mile)	1062	1267	1553	1716	2043	2452
Running, 5 mph (12 min mile)	472	563	690	763	908	1089
Running, 5.2 mph (11.5 min mile)	531	633	776	858	1021	1225
Running, 6 mph (10 min mile)	590	704	863	954	1135	1362
Running, 6.7 mph (9 min mile)	649	774	949	1049	1248	1498
Running, 7 mph (8.5 min mile)	679	809	992	1096	1305	1566
Running, 7.5mph (8 min mile)	738	880	1078	1192	1419	1703
Running, 8 mph (7.5 min mile)	797	950	1165	1287	1533	1839
Running, 8.6 mph (7 min mile)	826	985	1208	1335	1589	1907
Running, 9 mph (6.5 min mile)	885	1056	1294	1430	1703	2043
Running, cross country	531	633	776	858	1021	1225
Running, general	472	563	690	763	908	1089
Running, in place	472	563	690	763	908	1089
Running, on a track, team practice	590	704	863	954	1135	1362
Running, stairs, up	885	1056	1294	1430	1703	2043
Running, training, pushing wheelchair	472	563	690	763	908	1089
Running, wheeling, general	177	211	259	286	341	409
Sailing, boat/board, windsurfing, general	177	211	259	286	341	409
Sailing, in competition	295	352	431	477	567	681
Scrubbing floors, on hands and knees	325	387	474	524	624	749
Shoveling snow, by hand	354	422	518	572	681	817
Shuffleboard, lawn bowling	177	211	259	286	341	409
Sitting-playing with child(ren)-light	148	176	216	239	284	341
Skateboarding	295	352	431	477	567	681
Skating, ice, 9 mph or less	325	387	474	524	624	749
Skating, ice, general	413	493	604	668	795	954
Skating, ice, rapidly, > 9 mph	531	633	776	858	1021	1225
Skating, ice, speed, competitive	885	1056	1294	1430	1703	2043
Skating, roller	413	493	604	668	795	954
Ski jumping (climb up carrying skis)	413	493	604	668	795	954
Ski machine, general	561	669	819	906	1078	1294
Skiing, cross-country, >8.0 mph, racing	826	985	1208	1335	1589	1907

Activity Per Hour	Calories Burned by Weight in Pounds					
	130	155	190	210	250	300
Skiing, cross-country, moderate effort	472	563	690	763	908	1089
Skiing, cross-country, slow or light effort	413	493	604	668	795	954
Skiing, cross-country, uphill, maximum effort	974	1161	1423	1573	1873	2247
Skiing, cross-country, vigorous effort	531	633	776	858	1021	1225
Skiing, downhill, light effort	295	352	431	477	567	681
Skiing, downhill, moderate effort	354	422	518	572	681	817
Skiing, downhill, vigorous effort, racing	472	563	690	763	908	1089
Skiing, snow, general	413	493	604	668	795	954
Skiing, water	354	422	518	572	681	817
Ski-mobiling, water	413	493	604	668	795	954
Skin diving, scuba diving, general	413	493	604	668	795	954
Sledding, tobogganing, bobsledding, luge	413	493	604	668	795	954
Snorkeling	295	352	431	477	567	681
Snow shoeing	472	563	690	763	908	1089
Snowmobiling	207	246	302	334	397	477
Soccer, casual, general	413	493	604	668	795	954
Soccer, competitive	590	704	863	954	1135	1362
Softball or baseball, fast or slow pitch	295	352	431	477	567	681
Softball, officiating	354	422	518	572	681	817
Squash	708	844	1035	1144	1362	1634
Stair-treadmill ergometer, general	354	422	518	572	681	817
Standing-packing/unpacking boxes	207	246	302	334	397	477
Stretching, hatha yoga	236	281	345	381	454	544
Surfing, body or board	177	211	259	286	341	409
Sweeping garage, sidewalk	236	281	345	381	454	544
Swimming laps, freestyle, fast, vigorous effort	590	704	863	954	1135	1362
Swimming laps, freestyle, light/moderate effort	472	563	690	763	908	1089
Swimming, backstroke, general	472	563	690	763	908	1089
Swimming, breaststroke, general	590	704	863	954	1135	1362
Swimming, butterfly, general	649	774	949	1049	1248	1498
Swimming, leisurely, general	354	422	518	572	681	817
Swimming, sidestroke, general	472	563	690	763	908	1089
Swimming, sychronized	472	563	690	763	908	1089
Swimming, treading water, fast/vigorous	590	704	863	954	1135	1362
Swimming, treading water, moderate effort	236	281	345	381	454	544
Table tennis, ping pong	236	281	345	381	454	544

Calories Burned by Weight in Pounds

Activity Per Hour	130	155	190	210	250	300
Tai chi	236	281	345	381	454	544
Teaching aerobics class	354	422	518	572	681	817
Tennis, doubles	354	422	518	572	681	817
Tennis, general	413	493	604	668	795	954
Tennis, singles	472	563	690	763	908	1089
Unicycling	295	352	431	477	567	681
Volleyball, beach	472	563	690	763	908	1089
Volleyball, competitive, in gymnasium	236	281	345	381	454	544
Volleyball, noncompetitive; 6-9 member team	177	211	259	286	341	409
Walk/run-playing with child(ren)-moderate	236	281	345	381	454	544
Walk/run-playing with child(ren)-vigorous	295	352	431	477	567	681
Walking, 2.0 mph, slow pace	148	176	216	239	284	341
Walking, 3.0 mph, mod. pace, walking dog	207	246	302	334	397	477
Walking, 3.5 mph, uphill	354	422	518	572	681	817
Walking, 4.0 mph, very brisk pace	236	281	345	381	454	544
Walking, carrying infant or 15-lb load	207	246	302	334	397	477
Walking, grass track	295	352	431	477	567	681
Walking, upstairs	472	563	690	763	908	1089
Walking, using crutches	236	281	345	381	454	544
Wallyball, general	413	493	604	668	795	954
Water aerobics, water calisthenics	236	281	345	381	454	544
Water polo	590	704	863	954	1135	1362
Water volleyball	177	211	259	286	341	409
Weight lifting or body building, vigorous effort	354	422	518	572	681	817
Weight lifting, light or moderate effort	177	211	259	286	341	409
Whitewater rafting, kayaking, or canoeing	295	352	431	477	567	681

Bibliography

"109th U.S. Congress (2005–2006) H.R. 554: 109th U.S. Congress (2005–2006) H.R. 554: Personal Responsibility in Food Consumption Act of 2005". GovTrack.us. http://www.govtrack.us/congress/bill.xpd?bill=h109-554. Retrieved 2008-07-24.

"Alabama "Obesity Penalty" Stirs Debate". Don Fernandez. http://www.webmd.com/diet/news/20080825/alabama-obesity-penalty-stirs-debate. Retrieved April 5, 2009.

"Anti-obesity drug no magic bullet". Canadian Broadcasting Corporation. January 2, 2007. http://www.cbc.ca/health/story/2007/01/02/rimonabant.html. Retrieved 2008-09-19.

"Diet composition and obesity among Canadian adults". Statistics Canada. http://www.statcan.gc.ca/pub/82-003-x/2009004/article/10933-eng.htm.

"Early Communication about an Ongoing Safety Review ofÂ Meridia (sibutramine hydrochloride)". FDA. http://www.fda.gov/Drugs/DrugSafety/PostmarketDrugSafetyInformationforPatientsandProviders/DrugSafetyInformationforHeathcareProfessionals/ucm191650.htm. Retrieved Nov 23, 2009.

"EarthTrends: Nutrition: Calorie supply per capita". World Resources Institute. http://earthtrends.wri.org/searchable_db/index.php?theme=8&variable_ID=212&action=select_countries. Retrieved Oct. 18, 2009.

"FAO: Food Security Statistics". Food and Agriculture Organization of the United Nations. http://www.fao.org/economic/ess/food-security-statistics/en/. Retrieved Oct. 18, 2009.

"FDA Briefing Document NDA 21-888 Zimulti (rimonabant) Tablets, 20 mg Sanofi Aventis Advisory Committee" (PDF). Food and Drug Administration. June 13, 2007. http://www.fda.gov/ohrms/dockets/ac/07/briefing/2007-4306b1-fda-backgrounder.pdf. Retrieved 2008-09-19.

"Fewer Sugary Drinks Key to Weight Loss - healthfinder.gov". U.S. Department of Health and Human Services. http://www.healthfinder.gov/news/newsstory.aspx?docID=625759. Retrieved Oct 18,2009.

"Global Prevalence of Adult Obesity" (PDF). International Obesity Taskforce. http://www.iotf.org/database/documents/GlobalPrevalenceofAdultObesity16thDecember08.pdf. Retrieved January 29, 2008.

"Healthy Weight: Assessing Your Weight: BMI: About BMI for Children and Teens". Center for disease control and prevention http://www.cdc.gov/nccdphp/dnpa/healthyweight/assessing/bmi/childrens_BMI/about_childrens_BMI.htm. Retrieved April 6, 2009

"History of Medicine: Sushruta – the Clinician – Teacher par Excellence" (PDF). Dwivedi, Girish & Dwivedi, Shridhar. 2007. http://medind.nic.in/iae/t07/i4/iaet07i4p243.pdf. Retrieved 2008-09-19.

"International Size Acceptance Association – ISAA". International Size Acceptance Association. http://www.size-acceptance.org/. Retrieved January 13, 2009.

"ISAA Mission Statement". International Size Acceptance Association. http://www.size-acceptance.org/mission.html. Retrieved February 17, 2009.

"Media + Child and Adolescent Health: A Systematic Review" (pdf). Ezekiel J. Emanuel. Common Sense Media. 2008. http://www.commonsensemedia.org/sites/default/files/CSM_media+health_v2c%20110708.pdf. Retrieved April 6, 2009.

"Meridia (sibutramine hydrochloride): Follow-Up to an Early Communication about an Ongoing Safety Review". http://www.fda.gov/Safety/MedWatch/SafetyInformation/SafetyAlertsforHumanMedicalProducts/ucm198221.htm.

"Metabolism alone doesn't explain how thin people stay thin" (registration required). John Schieszer. The Medical Post. http://www.medicalpost.com/therapeutics/nutrition/article.jsp?content=20080818_121920_25640. Retrieved December 31, 2008.

"Obesity and Overweight" (PDF). World Health Organization. http://www.who.int/dietphysicalactivity/media/en/gsfs_obesity.pdf. Retrieved February 22, 2009.

"Obesity and overweight". World Health Organization. http://www.who.int/mediacentre/factsheets/fs311/en/index.html. Retrieved April 8th, 2009.

"Obesity and overweight: Economic consequences". Centers for Disease Control and Prevention. http://www.cdc.gov/nccdphp/dnpa/obesity/economic_consequences.htm. Retrieved 2007-09-05.

"Obesity Guidelines Website". Australian Government Department of Health and Ageing. http://www.health.gov.au/internet/main/publishing.nsf/Content/obesityguidelines-index.htm. Retrieved Oct. 25, 2009.

"Obesity, n". Oxford English Dictionary 2008. http://www.oed.com/. Retrieved March 21, 2009.

"Obesity: guidance on the prevention, identification, assessment and management of overweight and obesity in adults and children" (pdf). National Institute for Health and Clinical Excellence(NICE). National Health Services (NHS). 2006. http://www.nice.org.uk/nicemedia/pdf/CG43NICEGuideline.pdf. Retrieved April 8th,2009.

"Obesity: Time bomb or dud?". USA Today. 2005-05-25. http://www.usatoday.com/news/health/2005-05-25-obesity_x.htm. Retrieved 2008-09-21.

"Online Etymology Dictionary: Obesity". Douglas Harper. http://www.etymonline.com/index.php?term=obesity. Retrieved December 31, 2008.

"USDA: frsept99b". United States Department of Agriculture. http://www.scribd.com/doc/1470965/USDA-frsept99b. Retrieved January 10, 2009.

"What is NAAFA". National Association to Advance Fat Acceptance. http://www.capitalnaafa.org/whatisnaafa.html. Retrieved February 17, 2009.

"WHO | Physical Inactivity: A Global Public Health Problem". World Health Organization. http://www.who.int/dietphysicalactivity/factsheet_inactivity/en/index.html. Retrieved February 22, 2009.

"WHO: Obesity and overweight". World Health Organization. http://www.who.int/dietphysicalactivity/publications/facts/obesity/en/. Retrieved January 10, 2009.

"WIN – Publication – Prescription Medications for the Treatment of Obesity". National Institute of Diabetes and Digestive and Kidney Diseases (NIDDK). National Institutes of Health. http://win.niddk.nih.gov/publications/prescription.htm#fdameds. Retrieved January 14, 2009.

"www.paho.org". Pan American Health Organization. http://www.paho.org/English/DD/PIN/ePersp001_article01.htm. Retrieved January 10, 2009.

^ Christakis NA, Fowler JH (2007). "The Spread of Obesity in a Large Social Network over 32 Years". New England Journal of Medicine 357 (4): 370–379. doi:10.1056/NEJMsa066082. PMID 17652652.

(PDF) Storing up problems; the medical case for a slimmer nation. London: Royal College of Physicians. 2004-02-11. ISBN 1-86016-200-2. http://www.rcplondon.ac.uk/pubs/contents/ca4032bf-7b10-4e2f-8701-b24874f84514.pdf.

Adams JP, Murphy PG (July 2000). "Obesity in anaesthesia and intensive care". Br J Anaesth 85 (1): 91–108. doi:10.1093/bja/85.1.91. PMID 10927998. http://bja.oxfordjournals.org/cgi/content/full/85/1/91.

Adams TD, Gress RE, Smith SC, et al. (2007). "Long-term mortality after gastric bypass surgery". N. Engl. J. Med. 357 (8): 753–61. doi:10.1056/NEJMoa066603. PMID 17715409.

Allison DB, Fontaine KR, Manson JE, Stevens J, VanItallie TB (October 1999). "Annual deaths attributable to obesity in the United States". JAMA 282 (16): 1530–8. doi:10.1001/jama.282.16.1530. PMID 10546692. http://jama.ama-assn.org/cgi/content/full/282/16/1530.

Anand G, Katz PO (2008). "Gastroesophageal reflux disease and obesity". Rev Gastroenterol Disord 8 (4): 233–9. PMID 19107097. http://www.medreviews.com/pubmed.cfm?j=3&v=8&i=4&p=233.

Anderson JW, Konz EC, Frederich RC, Wood CL (1 November 2001). "Long-term weight-loss maintenance: A meta-analysis of US studies". Am. J. Clin. Nutr. 74 (5): 579–84. PMID 11684524. http://www.ajcn.org/cgi/content/full/74/5/579.

Arendas K, Qiu Q, Gruslin A (June 2008). "Obesity in pregnancy: pre-conceptional to postpartum consequences". J Obstet Gynaecol Can 30 (6): 477–88. PMID 18611299.

Areton (January 2002). "Factors in the sexual satisfaction of obese women in relationships". Electronic Journal of Human Sexuality 5. http://www.ejhs.org/volume5/Areton/06Partners.htm.

Bakewell J (2007). "Bariatric furniture: Considerations for use.". Int J Ther Rehabil (7): 329–33. http://www.ijtr.co.uk/cgi-bin/go.pl/library/article.cgi?uid=23858;article=IJTR_14_7_329_333.

Barness LA, Opitz JM, Gilbert-Barness E (December 2007). "Obesity: genetic, molecular, and environmental aspects". Am. J. Med. Genet. A 143A (24): 3016–34. doi:10.1002/ajmg.a.32035. PMID 18000969.

Baron M (November 2004). "Commercial weight-loss programs". Health Care Food Nutr Focus 21 (11): 8–9. PMID 15559885. http://meta.wkhealth.com/pt/pt-core/template-journal/lwwgateway/media/landingpage.htm?issn=1090-2260&volume=21&issue=11&spage=8.

Bei-Fan Z; Cooperative Meta-Analysis Group of Working Group on Obesity in China (December 2002). "Predictive values of body mass index and waist circumference for risk factors of certain related diseases in Chinese adults: study on optimal cut-off points of body mass index and waist circumference in Chinese adults". Asia Pac J Clin Nutr 11 Suppl 8: S685–93. doi:10.1046/j.1440-6047.11.s8.9.x. PMID 12534691.

Bellows-Riecken KH, Rhodes RE (February 2008). "A birth of inactivity? A review of physical activity and parenthood". Prev Med 46 (2): 99–110. doi:10.1016/j.ypmed.2007.08.003. PMID 17919713.

Bessesen DH (June 2008). "Update on obesity". J. Clin. Endocrinol. Metab. 93 (6): 2027–34. doi:10.1210/jc.2008-0520. PMID 18539769.

Beydoun MA, Beydoun HA, Wang Y (May 2008). "Obesity and central obesity as risk factors for incident dementia and its subtypes: A systematic review and meta-analysis". Obes Rev 9 (3): 204–18. doi:10.1111/j.1467-789X.2008.00473.x. PMID 18331422.

Bigal ME, Lipton RB (January 2008). "Obesity and chronic daily headache". Curr Pain Headache Rep 12 (1): 56–61. doi:10.1007/s11916-008-0011-8. PMID 18417025.

Bjornstop P (2001). "Do stress reactions cause abdominal obesity and comorbidities?". Obesity Reviews 2 (2): 73–86. doi:10.1046/j.1467-789x.2001.00027.x. PMID 12119665.

Bleich S, Cutler D, Murray C, Adams A (2008). "Why is the developed world obese?". Annu Rev Public Health 29: 273–95. doi:10.1146/annurev.publhealth.29.020907.090954. PMID 18173389.

Borodulin K, Laatikainen T, Juolevi A, Jousilahti P (June 2008). "Thirty-year trends of physical activity in relation to age, calendar time and birth cohort in Finnish adults". Eur J Public Health 18 (3): 339–44. doi:10.1093/eurpub/ckm092. PMID 17875578.

Boss, Olivier; Karl G. Hofbauer (2004). Pharmacotherapy of obesity: options and alternatives. Boca Raton: CRC Press. pp. 286. ISBN 0-415-30321-4. http://books.google.ca/books?id=v7o5e8aSXB0C&pg=PA286&lpg=PA286&dq=Amphetamines+are+not+FDA+approved+to+treat+obesity&source=web&ots=6pX54AHIK-&sig=eQOKZW0RA6xuZvsd3G5GG_aCc38&hl=en&sa=X&oi=book_result&resnum=5&ct=result#PPA286,M1. Retrieved January 14, 2009.

Boulpaep, Emile L.; Boron, Walter F. (2003). Medical physiologya: A cellular and molecular approach. Philadelphia: Saunders. pp. 1227. ISBN 0-7216-3256-4.

Bravata DM, Smith-Spangler C, Sundaram V, et al. (November 2007). "Using pedometers to increase physical activity and improve health: a systematic review". JAMA : the journal of the American Medical Association 298 (19): 2296–304. doi:10.1001/jama.298.19.2296. PMID 18029834.

Bray GA (2004). "Medical consequences of obesity". J. Clin. Endocrinol. Metab. 89 (6): 2583–9. doi:10.1210/jc.2004-0535. PMID 15181027.

Brennan Ramirez LK, Hoehner CM, Brownson RC et al. (December 2006). "Indicators of activity-friendly communities: An evidence-based consensus process". Am J Prev Med 31 (6): 530–32. doi:10.1016/j.amepre.2006.07.026. PMID 17169714.

Breslow L (September 1952). "Public health aspects of weight control". Am J Public Health Nations Health 42 (9): 1116–20. PMID 12976585.

Brook Barnes (2007-07-18). "Limiting Ads of Junk Food to Children". New York Times. http://www.nytimes.com/2007/07/18/business/18food.html. Retrieved 2008-07-24.

Brownson RC, Boehmer TK, Luke DA (2005). "Declining rates of physical activity in the United States: what are the contributors?". Annu Rev Public Health 26: 421–43. doi:10.1146/annurev.publhealth.26.021304.144437. PMID 15760296.

Caballero B (2007). "The global epidemic of obesity: An overview". Epidemiol Rev 29: 1–5. doi:10.1093/epirev/mxm012. PMID 17569676.

Caballero B (March 2001). "Introduction. Symposium: Obesity in developing countries: biological and ecological factors". J. Nutr. 131 (3): 866S–870S. PMID 11238776. http://jn.nutrition.org/cgi/content/full/131/3/866S.

Calle EE, Rodriguez C, Walker-Thurmond K, Thun MJ (April 2003). "Overweight, obesity, and mortality from cancer in a prospectively studied cohort of U.S. adults". N. Engl. J. Med. 348 (17): 1625–38. doi:10.1056/NEJMoa021423. PMID 12711737.

Calle EE, Thun MJ, Petrelli JM, Rodriguez C, Heath CW (October 1999). "Body-mass index and mortality in a prospective cohort of U.S. adults". N. Engl. J. Med. 341 (15): 1097–105. doi:10.1056/NEJM199910073411501. PMID 10511607. http://content.nejm.org/cgi/content/full/341/15/1097.

Campos, Paul F. (2005). The Diet Myth. Gotham. pp. xiv,xvii. ISBN 1-59240-135-X.

Chakravarthy MV, Booth FW (2004). "Eating, exercise, and "thrifty" genotypes: Connecting the dots toward an evolutionary understanding of modern chronic diseases". J. Appl. Physiol. 96 (1): 3–10. doi:10.1152/japplphysiol.00757.2003. PMID 14660491.

Chiles C, van Wattum PJ. Psychiatric aspects of the obesity crisis. Psychiatr Times. 2010;27(4):47-51.

Chiolero A, Faeh D, Paccaud F, Cornuz J (1 April 2008). "Consequences of smoking for body weight, body fat distribution, and insulin resistance". Am. J. Clin. Nutr. 87 (4): 801–9. PMID 18400700. http://www.ajcn.org/cgi/content/full/87/4/801.

Choi HK, Atkinson K, Karlson EW, Curhan G (April 2005). "Obesity, weight change, hypertension, diuretic use, and risk of gout in men: the health professionals follow-up study". Arch. Intern. Med. 165 (7): 742–8. doi:10.1001/archinte.165.7.742. PMID 15824292.

Cohen PA, McCormick D, Casey C, Dawson GF, Hacker KA (December 2007). "Imported Compounded Diet Pill Use Among Brazilian Women Immigrants in the United States". J Immigr Minor Health 11 (3): 229–36. doi:10.1007/s10903-007-9099-x. PMID 18066718.

Cummings, Laura (5 February 2003). "The diet business: Banking on failure". BBC News. http://news.bbc.co.uk/2/hi/business/2725943.stm. Retrieved 25 February 2009.

Dannenberg AL, Burton DC, Jackson RJ (2004). "Economic and environmental costs of obesity: The impact on airlines". American journal of preventive medicine 27 (3): 264. doi:10.1016/j.amepre.2004.06.004. PMID 15450642.

Darvall KA, Sam RC, Silverman SH, Bradbury AW, Adam DJ (February 2007). "Obesity and thrombosis". Eur J Vasc Endovasc Surg 33 (2): 223–33. doi:10.1016/j.ejvs.2006.10.006. PMID 17185009.

Dentali F, Squizzato A, Ageno W (July 2009). "The metabolic syndrome as a risk factor for venous and arterial thrombosis". Semin. Thromb. Hemost. 35 (5): 451–7. doi:10.1055/s-0029-1234140. PMID 19739035.

Di Castelnuovo A, Quacquaruccio G, Donati MB, de Gaetano G, Iacoviello L (January 2009). "Spousal concordance for major coronary risk factors: a systematic review and meta-analysis". Am. J. Epidemiol. 169 (1): 1–8. doi:10.1093/aje/kwn234. PMID 18845552.

DiBaise JK, Zhang H, Crowell MD, Krajmalnik-Brown R, Decker GA, Rittmann BE (April 2008). "Gut microbiota and its possible relationship with obesity". Mayo Clinic proceedings. Mayo Clinic 83 (4): 460–9. doi:10.4065/83.4.460. PMID 18380992.

Diercks DB, Roe MT, Mulgund J et al. (July 2006). "The obesity paradox in non-ST-segment elevation acute coronary syndromes: Results from the Can Rapid risk stratification of Unstable angina patients Suppress ADverse outcomes with Early implementation of the American College of Cardiology/American Heart Association Guidelines Quality Improvement Initiative". Am Heart J 152 (1): 140–8. doi:10.1016/j.ahj.2005.09.024. PMID 16824844.

Dollman J, Norton K, Norton L (December 2005). "Evidence for secular trends in children's physical activity behaviour". Br J Sports Med 39 (12): 892–7; discussion 897. doi:10.1136/bjsm.2004.016675. PMID 16306494.

Douglas Martin (1991-07-31). "About New York". New York Times. http://www.nytimes.com/1991/07/31/nyregion/about-new-york.html. Retrieved 2008-07-24.

Drewnowski A, Specter SE (January 2004). "Poverty and obesity: the role of energy density and energy costs". Am. J. Clin. Nutr. 79 (1): 6–16. PMID 14684391. http://www.ajcn.org/cgi/content/full/79/1/6.

Ejerblad E, Fored CM, Lindblad P, Fryzek J, McLaughlin JK, Nyrén O (2006). "Obesity and risk for chronic renal failure". J. Am. Soc. Nephrol. 17 (6): 1695–702. doi:10.1681/ASN.2005060638. PMID 16641153.

Encinosa WE, Bernard DM, Chen CC, Steiner CA (2006). "Healthcare utilization and outcomes after bariatric surgery". Medical care 44 (8): 706–12. doi:10.1097/01.mlr.0000220833.89050.ed. PMID 16862031.

Esposito K, Giugliano F, Di Palo C, Giugliano G, Marfella R, D'Andrea F, D'Armiento M, Giugliano D (2004). "Effect of lifestyle changes on erectile dysfunction in obese men: A randomized controlled trial". JAMA 291 (24): 2978–84. doi:10.1001/jama.291.24.2978. PMID 15213209.

Falagas ME, Kompoti M (July 2006). "Obesity and infection". Lancet Infect Dis 6 (7): 438–46. doi:10.1016/S1473-3099(06)70523-0. PMID 16790384.

Farooqi S, O'Rahilly S (December 2006). "Genetics of obesity in humans". Endocr. Rev. 27 (7): 710–18. doi:10.1210/er.2006-0040. PMID 17122358. http://edrv.endojournals.org/cgi/content/full/27/7/710.

Finkelstein EA, Fiebelkorn IA, Wang G (1 January 2003). "National medical spending attributable to overweight and obesity: How much, and who's paying". Health Affairs Online (May). http://content.healthaffairs.org/cgi/content/full/hlthaff.w3.219v1/DC1.

Flanagan CM, Kaesberg JL, Mitchell ES, Ferguson MA, Haigney MC (August 2008). "Coronary artery aneurysm and thrombosis following chronic ephedra use". Int. J. Cardiol. 139 (1): e11–3. doi:10.1016/j.ijcard.2008.06.081. PMID 18718687.

Flegal KM, Carroll MD, Ogden CL, Johnson CL (October 2002). "Prevalence and trends in obesity among US adults, 1999–2000". JAMA 288 (14): 1723–1727. doi:10.1001/jama.288.14.1723. PMID 12365955. http://jama.ama-assn.org/cgi/content/full/288/14/1723.

Flegal KM, Ogden CL, Wei R, Kuczmarski RL, Johnson CL (June 2001). "Prevalence of overweight in US children: comparison of US growth charts from the Centers for Disease Control and Prevention with other reference values for body mass index". Am. J. Clin. Nutr. 73 (6): 1086–93. PMID 11382664. http://www.ajcn.org/cgi/content/full/73/6/1086.

Flegal KM, Troiano RP, Pamuk ER, Kuczmarski RJ, Campbell SM (November 1995). "The influence of smoking cessation on the prevalence of overweight in the United States". N.

Engl. J. Med. 333 (18): 1165–70. doi:10.1056/NEJM199511023331801. PMID 7565970. http://content.nejm.org/cgi/content/full/333/18/1165.

Flier JS (2004). "Obesity wars: Molecular progress confronts an expanding epidemic". Cell 116 (2): 337–50. doi:10.1016/S0092-8674(03)01081-X. PMID 14744442.

Flynn MA, McNeil DA, Maloff B, et al. (February 2006). "Reducing obesity and related chronic disease risk in children and youth: a synthesis of evidence with 'best practice' recommendations". Obes Rev 7 Suppl 1: 7–66. doi:10.1111/j.1467-789X.2006.00242.x. PMID 16371076.

Fonseca V (2003). "Effect of thiazolidinediones on body weight in patients with diabetes mellitus". Am. J. Med. 115 Suppl 8A: 42S–48S. doi:10.1016/j.amjmed.2003.09.005. PMID 14678865.

Freedman DM, Ron E, Ballard-Barbash R, Doody MM, Linet MS (May 2006). "Body mass index and all-cause mortality in a nationwide US cohort". Int J Obes (Lond) 30 (5): 822–9. doi:10.1038/sj.ijo.0803193. PMID 16404410.

Fried M, Hainer V, Basdevant A, et al. (April 2007). "Inter-disciplinary European guidelines on surgery of severe obesity". Int J Obes (Lond) 31 (4): 569–77. doi:10.1038/sj.ijo.0803560. PMID 17325689.

Fumento, Michael (1997). The Fat of the Land: Our Health Crisis and How Overweight Americans Can Help Themselves. Penguin (Non-Classics). pp. 126. ISBN 0-14-026144-3.

Gard, Michael (2005). The Obesity Epidemic: Science, Morality and Ideology. Routledge. pp. 15 and 153. ISBN 0415318963.

Giugliano G, Nicoletti G, Grella E, et al. (April 2004). "Effect of liposuction on insulin resistance and vascular inflammatory markers in obese women". Br J Plast Surg 57 (3): 190–4. doi:10.1016/j.bjps.2003.12.010. PMID 15006519.

Goodman E, Adler NE, Daniels SR, Morrison JA, Slap GB, Dolan LM (2003). "Impact of objective and subjective social status on obesity in a biracial cohort of adolescents". Obesity Reviews 11 (8): 1018–26. doi:10.1038/oby.2003.140.

Gortmaker SL, Must A, Sobol AM, Peterson K, Colditz GA, Dietz WH (April 1996). "Television viewing as a cause of increasing obesity among children in the United States, 1986–1990". Arch Pediatr Adolesc Med 150 (4): 356–62. PMID 8634729.

Gray DS, Fujioka K (1991). "Use of relative weight and Body Mass Index for the determination of adiposity". J Clin Epidemiol 44 (6): 545–50. doi:10.1016/0895-4356(91)90218-X. PMID 2037859.

Great Britain Parliament House of Commons Health Committee (May 2004). Obesity – Volume 1 – HCP 23-I, Third Report of session 2003–04. Report, together with formal minutes. London, UK: TSO (The Stationery Office). ISBN status=May be invalid – please double check. http://www.publications.parliament.uk/pa/cm200304/cmselect/cmhealth/23/2302.htm. Retrieved 2007-12-17.

Grundy SM (2004). "Obesity, metabolic syndrome, and cardiovascular disease". J. Clin. Endocrinol. Metab. 89 (6): 2595–600. doi:10.1210/jc.2004-0372. PMID 15181029.

Gwinup G (1987). "Weight loss without dietary restriction: Efficacy of different forms of aerobic exercise". Am J Sports Med 15 (3): 275–9. doi:10.1177/036354658701500317. PMID 3618879.

Habbu A, Lakkis NM, Dokainish H (October 2006). "The obesity paradox: Fact or fiction?". Am. J. Cardiol. 98 (7): 944–8. doi:10.1016/j.amjcard.2006.04.039. PMID 16996880.

Hahler B (June 2006). "An overview of dermatological conditions commonly associated with the obese patient". Ostomy Wound Manage 52 (6): 34–6, 38, 40 passim. PMID 16799182.

Hamann A, Matthaei S (1996). "Regulation of energy balance by leptin". Exp. Clin. Endocrinol. Diabetes 104 (4): 293–300. doi:10.1055/s-0029-1211457. PMID 8886745.

Harney D, Patijn J (2007). "Meralgia paresthetica: diagnosis and management strategies". Pain Med 8 (8): 669–77. doi:10.1111/j.1526-4637.2006.00227.x. PMID 18028045.

Haskell WL, Lee IM, Pate RR, et al. (August 2007). "Physical activity and public health: updated recommendation for adults from the American College of Sports Medicine and the American Heart Association". Circulation 116 (9): 1081–93. doi:10.1161/CIRCULATIONAHA.107.185649. PMID 17671237.

Haslam D (March 2007). "Obesity: a medical history". Obes Rev 8 Suppl 1: 31–6. doi:10.1111/j.1467-789X.2007.00314.x. PMID 17316298.

Heshka S, Anderson JW, Atkinson RL, et al. (April 2003). "Weight loss with self-help compared with a structured commercial program: a randomized trial". JAMA 289 (14): 1792–8. doi:10.1001/jama.289.14.1792. PMID 12684357.

Hewitt, Duncan (May 23, 2000). "China battles obesity". BBC. http://news.bbc.co.uk/2/hi/health/760787.stm. Retrieved August 8, 2009.

Howard, Natasha J.; Taylor, A; Gill, T; Chittleborough, C (March 2008). "Severe obesity: Investigating the socio-demographics within the extremes of body mass index". Obesity Research &Clinical Practice 2 (1): 51–59. doi:10.1016/j.orcp.2008.01.001.

Hunskaar S (2008). "A systematic review of overweight and obesity as risk factors and targets for clinical intervention for urinary incontinence in women". Neurourol. Urodyn. 27 (8): 749–57. doi:10.1002/nau.20635. PMID 18951445.

Imaz I, Martínez-Cervell C, García-Alvarez EE, Sendra-Gutiérrez JM, González-Enríquez J (July 2008). "Safety and effectiveness of the intragastric balloon for obesity. A meta-analysis". Obes Surg 18 (7): 841–6. doi:10.1007/s11695-007-9331-8. PMID 18459025.

James WP (March 2008). "The fundamental drivers of the obesity epidemic". Obes Rev 9 Suppl 1: 6–13. doi:10.1111/j.1467-789X.2007.00432.x. PMID 18307693.

Johnson F, Cooke L, Croker H, Wardle J (2008). "Changing perceptions of weight in Great Britain: comparison of two population surveys". BMJ 337: a494. doi:10.1136/bmj.a494. PMID 18617488. PMC 2500200. http://www.bmj.com/cgi/content/full/337/jul10_1/a494.

Kahn EB, Ramsey LT, Brownson RC, et al. (May 2002). "The effectiveness of interventions to increase physical activity. A systematic review". Am J Prev Med 22 (4 Suppl): 73–107. doi:10.1016/S0749-3797(02)00434-8. PMID 11985936.

Kanazawa M, Yoshiike N, Osaka T, Numba Y, Zimmet P, Inoue S (December 2002). "Criteria and classification of obesity in Japan and Asia-Oceania". Asia Pac J Clin Nutr 11 Suppl 8: S732–S737. doi:10.1046/j.1440-6047.11.s8.19.x. PMID 12534701.

Keith SW, Redden DT, Katzmarzyk PT, et al. (2006). "Putative contributors to the secular increase in obesity: Exploring the roads less traveled". Int J Obes (Lond) 30 (11): 1585–94. doi:10.1038/sj.ijo.0803326. PMID 16801930. http://www.nature.com/ijo/journal/v30/n11/full/0803326a.html.

Klein S, Fontana L, Young VL, et al. (June 2004). "Absence of an effect of liposuction on insulin action and risk factors for coronary heart disease". N. Engl. J. Med. 350 (25): 2549–57. doi:10.1056/NEJMoa033179. PMID 15201411.

Kolata,Gina (2007). Rethinking thin: The new science of weight loss – and the myths and realities of dieting. Picador. pp. 122. ISBN 0-312-42785-9.

Kushner, Robert (2007). Treatment of the Obese Patient (Contemporary Endocrinology). Totowa, NJ: Humana Press. pp. 158. ISBN 1-59745

Lau DC, Douketis JD, Morrison KM, Hramiak IM, Sharma AM, Ur E (April 2007). "2006 Canadian clinical practice guidelines on the management and prevention of obesity in adults and children [summary"]. CMAJ 176 (8): S1–13. doi:10.1503/cmaj.061409. PMID 17420481.

Lau DC, Douketis JD, Morrison KM, Hramiak IM, Sharma AM, Ur E (April 2007). "2006 Canadian clinical practice guidelines on the management and prevention of obesity in adults and children [summary]". CMAJ 176 (8): S1–13. doi:10.1503/cmaj.061409. PMID 17420481. PMC 1839777. http://www.cmaj.ca/cgi/content/full/176/8/S1.

Lee L, Kumar S, Leong LC (February 1994). "The impact of five-month basic military training on the body weight and body fat of 197 moderately to severely obese Singaporean males aged 17 to 19 years". Int. J. Obes. Relat. Metab. Disord. 18 (2): 105–9. PMID 8148923.

Li Z, Maglione M, Tu W, et al. (April 2005). "Meta-analysis: pharmacologic treatment of obesity". Ann. Intern. Med. 142 (7): 532–46. PMID 15809465. http://www.annals.org/cgi/content/full/142/7/532.

Lin BH, Guthrie J and Frazao E (1999). "Nutrient contribution of food away from home". in Frazão E. Agriculture Information Bulletin No. 750: America's Eating Habits: Changes and Consequences. Washington, DC: US Department of Agriculture, Economic Research Service. pp. 213–239. http://www.ers.usda.gov/publications/aib750/.

Lisa DiCarlo (2002-10-24). "Why Airlines Can't Cut The Fat". Forbes.com. http://www.forbes.com/2002/10/24/cx_ld_1024obese.html. Retrieved 2008-07-23.

Loscalzo, Joseph; Fauci, Anthony S.; Braunwald, Eugene; Dennis L. Kasper; Hauser, Stephen L; Longo, Dan L. (2008). Harrison's principles of internal medicine. McGraw-Hill Medical. ISBN 0-07-146633-9.

Lund Elizabeth M. (2006). "Prevalence and Risk Factors for Obesity in Adult Dogs from Private US Veterinary Practices". Intern J Appl Res Vet Med 4 (2): 177–86. http://www.jarvm.com/articles/Vol4Iss2/Lund.pdf.

MacLeod, Calum (August 1, 2007). "Obesity of China's kids stuns officials". USA Today. http://www.usatoday.com/news/world/2007-01-08-chinese-obesity_x.htm. Retrieved August 8, 2009.

Makhsida N, Shah J, Yan G, Fisch H, Shabsigh R (September 2005). "Hypogonadism and metabolic syndrome: Implications for testosterone therapy". J. Urol. 174 (3): 827–34. doi:10.1097/01.ju.0000169490.78443.59. PMID 16093964.

Malik VS, Schulze MB, Hu FB (August 2006). "Intake of sugar-sweetened beverages and weight gain: a systematic review". Am. J. Clin. Nutr. 84 (2): 274–88. PMID 16895873. http://www.ajcn.org/cgi/content/full/84/2/274.

Manson JE, Willett WC, Stampfer MJ, et al. (1995). "Body weight and mortality among women". N. Engl. J. Med. 333 (11): 677–85. doi:10.1056/NEJM199509143331101. PMID 7637744.

Marantz PR, Bird ED, Alderman MH (March 2008). "A call for higher standards of evidence for dietary guidelines". Am J Prev Med 34 (3): 234–40. doi:10.1016/j.amepre.2007.11.017. PMID 18312812.

Mary Jones. "Case Study: Cataplexy and SOREMPs Without Excessive Daytime Sleepiness in Prader Willi Syndrome. Is This the Beginning of Narcolepsy in a Five Year Old?". European Society of Sleep Technologists. http://www.esst.org/newsletter2000.htm. Retrieved April 6, 2009.

McGreevy PD, Thomson PC, Pride C, Fawcett A, Grassi T, Jones B (May 2005). "Prevalence of obesity in dogs examined by Australian veterinary practices and the risk factors involved". Vet. Rec. 156 (22): 695–702. PMID 15923551.

McLaren L (2007). "Socioeconomic status and obesity". Epidemiol Rev 29: 29–48. doi:10.1093/epirev/mxm001. PMID 17478442.

Mokdad AH, Marks JS, Stroup DF, Gerberding JL (March 2004). "Actual causes of death in the United States, 2000" (PDF). JAMA 291 (10): 1238–45. doi:10.1001/jama.291.10.1238. PMID 15010446. http://www.csdp.org/research/1238.pdf.

Molenaar EA, Numans ME, van Ameijden EJ, Grobbee DE (November 2008). "[Considerable comorbidity in overweight adults: results from the Utrecht Health Project]" (in Dutch; Flemish). Ned Tijdschr Geneeskd 152 (45): 2457–63. PMID 19051798.

Munger KL, Chitnis T, Ascherio A. (2009). Body size and risk of MS in two cohorts of US women. Neurology. 73(19):1543-50. doi:10.1212/WNL.0b013e3181c0d6e0 PMID 19901245

National Association to Advance Fat Acceptance (2008), We come in all sizes, NAAFA, http://www.naafaonline.com/dev2/, retrieved 2008-07-29

National Control for Health Statistics. "Nutrition For Everyone". Centers for Disease Control and Prevention. http://www.cdc.gov/nccdphp/dnpa/nutrition/nutrition_for_everyone. Retrieved 2008-07-09.

National Heart, Lung, and Blood Institute (1998) (PDF). Clinical Guidelines on the Identification, Evaluation, and Treatment of Overweight and Obesity in Adults. International Medical Publishing, Inc. ISBN 1-58808-002-1. http://www.nhlbi.nih.gov/guidelines/obesity/ob_gdlns.pdf.

Neovius K, Johansson K, Kark M, Neovius M (January 2009). "Obesity status and sick leave: a systematic review". Obes Rev 10 (1): 17–27. doi:10.1111/j.1467-789X.2008.00521.x. PMID 18778315.

Ness-Abramof R, Apovian CM (February 2006). "Diet modification for treatment and prevention of obesity". Endocrine 29 (1): 5–9. doi:10.1385/ENDO:29:1:135. PMID 16622287.

Nestle M, Jacobson MF (2000). "Halting the obesity epidemic: A public health policy approach". Public Health Rep 115 (1): 12–24. doi:10.1093/phr/115.1.12. PMID 10968581.

Neumark-Sztainer D (March 1999). "The weight dilemma: a range of philosophical perspectives". Int. J. Obes. Relat. Metab. Disord. 23 Suppl 2: S31–7. doi:10.1038/sj.ijo.0800857. PMID 10340803.

Nijland ML, Stam F, Seidell JC (June 2009). "Overweight in dogs, but not in cats, is related to overweight in their owners". Public Health Nutr 13 (1): 1–5. doi:10.1017/S136898000999022X. PMID 19545467

Norris SL, Zhang X, Avenell A, Gregg E, Schmid CH, Lau J (2005). "Pharmacotherapy for weight loss in adults with type 2 diabetes mellitus". Cochrane database of systematic reviews (Online) (1): CD004096. doi:10.1002/14651858.CD004096.pub2. PMID 15674929.

Olsen NJ, Heitmann BL (January 2009). "Intake of calorically sweetened beverages and obesity". Obes Rev 10 (1): 68–75. doi:10.1111/j.1467-789X.2008.00523.x. PMID 18764885.

Oreopoulos A, Padwal R, Kalantar-Zadeh K, Fonarow GC, Norris CM, McAlister FA (July 2008). "Body mass index and mortality in heart failure: A meta-analysis". Am. Heart J. 156 (1): 13–22. doi:10.1016/j.ahj.2008.02.014. PMID 18585492.

Oreopoulos A, Padwal R, Norris CM, Mullen JC, Pretorius V, Kalantar-Zadeh K (February 2008). "Effect of obesity on short- and long-term mortality postcoronary revascularization: A meta-analysis". Obesity (Silver Spring) 16 (2): 442–50. doi:10.1038/oby.2007.36. PMID 18239657.

Ostbye T, Dement JM, Krause KM (2007). "Obesity and workers' compensation: Results from the Duke Health and Safety Surveillance System". Arch. Intern. Med. 167 (8): 766–73. doi:10.1001/archinte.167.8.766. PMID 17452538.

Peeters A, Barendregt JJ, Willekens F, Mackenbach JP, Al Mamun A, Bonneux L (January 2003). "Obesity in adulthood and its consequences for life expectancy: A life-table analysis" (PDF). Ann. Intern. Med. 138 (1): 24–32. PMID 12513041. http://www.annals.org/cgi/reprint/138/1/24.

Peeters A, O'Brien PE, Laurie C, et al. (December 2007). "Substantial intentional weight loss and mortality in the severely obese". Ann. Surg. 246 (6): 1028–33. doi:10.1097/SLA.0b013e31814a6929. PMID 18043106.

Pignone MP, Ammerman A, Fernandez L, et al. (2003). "Counseling to promote a healthy diet in adults: A summary of the evidence for the U.S. Preventive Services Task Force". American journal of preventive medicine 24 (1): 75–92. doi:10.1016/S0749-3797(02)00580-9. PMID 12554027.

Pischon T, Boeing H, Hoffmann K, et al. (November 2008). "General and abdominal adiposity and risk of death in Europe". N. Engl. J. Med. 359 (20): 2105–20. doi:10.1056/NEJMoa0801891. PMID 19005195.

Poirier P, Giles TD, Bray GA, et al. (May 2006). "Obesity and cardiovascular disease: pathophysiology, evaluation, and effect of weight loss". Arterioscler. Thromb. Vasc. Biol. 26 (5): 968–76. doi:10.1161/01.ATV.0000216787.85457.f3. PMID 16627822.

Pollan, Michael (22 April 2007). "You Are What You Grow". New York Times. http://www.nytimes.com/2007/04/22/magazine/22wwlnlede.t.html?ex=1186027200&en=bbe0f6a2c10e3b3c&ei=5070. Retrieved 2007-07-30.

Poobalan AS, Aucott LS, Smith WC, Avenell A, Jung R, Broom J (November 2007). "Long-term weight loss effects on all cause mortality in overweight/obese populations". Obes Rev 8 (6): 503–13. doi:10.1111/j.1467-789X.2007.00393.x. PMID 17949355.

Poulain M, Doucet M, Major GC, et al. (April 2006). "The effect of obesity on chronic respiratory diseases: pathophysiology and therapeutic strategies". CMAJ 174 (9): 1293–9. doi:10.1503/cmaj.051299. PMID 16636330. PMC 1435949. http://www.cmaj.ca/cgi/content/full/174/9/1293.

Puhl R, Brownell KD (December 2001). "Bias, discrimination, and obesity". Obes. Res. 9 (12): 788–805. doi:10.1038/oby.2001.108. PMID 11743063.

Puhl R., Henderson K., and Brownell K. 2005 p.29

Puhl R., Henderson K., and Brownell K. 2005 p.30

Pulver, Adam (2007). An Imperfect Fit: Obesity, Public Health, and Disability Anti-Discrimination Law. Social Science Electronic Publishing. http://papers.ssrn.com/sol3/papers.cfm?abstract_id=1316106. Retrieved January 13, 2009.

Rados C (2004). "Ephedra ban: no shortage of reasons". FDA Consum 38 (2): 6–7. PMID 15101356.

Romero-Corral A, Montori VM, Somers VK, et al. (2006). "Association of bodyweight with total mortality and with cardiovascular events in coronary artery disease: A systematic review of cohort studies". Lancet 368 (9536): 666–78. doi:10.1016/S0140-6736(06)69251-9. PMID 16920472.

Rosén T, Bosaeus I, Tölli J, Lindstedt G, Bengtsson BA (1993). "Increased body fat mass and decreased extracellular fluid volume in adults with growth hormone deficiency". Clin. Endocrinol. (Oxf) 38 (1): 63–71. doi:10.1111/j.1365-2265.1993.tb00974.x. PMID 8435887.

Rosenheck R (November 2008). "Fast food consumption and increased caloric intake: a systematic review of a trajectory towards weight gain and obesity risk". Obes Rev 9 (6): 535–47. doi:10.1111/j.1467-789X.2008.00477.x. PMID 18346099.

Rubinstein S, Caballero B (2000). "Is Miss America an undernourished role model?". JAMA 283 (12): 1569. doi:10.1001/jama.283.12.1569. PMID 10735392.

Rucker D, Padwal R, Li SK, Curioni C, Lau DC (2007). "Long term pharmacotherapy for obesity and overweight: Updated meta-analysis". BMJ 335 (7631): 1194–99. doi:10.1136/bmj.39385.413113.25. PMID 18006966. PMC 2128668. http://www.bmj.com/cgi/content/full/335/7631/1194.

Sacks FM, Bray GA, Carey VJ, et al. (February 2009). "Comparison of weight-loss diets with different compositions of fat, protein, and carbohydrates". N. Engl. J. Med. 360 (9): 859–73. doi:10.1056/NEJMoa0804748. PMID 19246357.

Sacks G, Swinburn B, Lawrence M (January 2009). "Obesity Policy Action framework and analysis grids for a comprehensive policy approach to reducing obesity". Obes Rev 10 (1): 76–86. doi:10.1111/j.1467-789X.2008.00524.x. PMID 18761640.

Sahlin K, Sallstedt EK, Bishop D, Tonkonogi M (December 2008). "Turning down lipid oxidation during heavy exercise—what is the mechanism?". J. Physiol. Pharmacol. 59 Suppl 7: 19–30. PMID 19258655. http://www.jpp.krakow.pl/journal/archive/1208_s7/pdf/19_1208_s7_article.pdf.

Salmon J, Timperio A (2007). "Prevalence, trends and environmental influences on child and youth physical activity". Med Sport Sci 50: 183–99. doi:10.1159/0000101391 (inactive 2009-10-31). PMID 17387258.

Satcher D (2001). The Surgeon General's Call to Action to Prevent and Decrease Overweight and Obesity. U.S. Dept. of Health and Human Services, Public Health Service, Office of Surgeon General. ISBN status=May be invalid – please double check. http://www.ncbi.nlm.nih.gov/bookshelf/br.fcgi?book=hssurggen&part=A2.

Schmidt DS, Salahudeen AK (2007). "Obesity-survival paradox-still a controversy?". Semin Dial 20 (6): 486–92. doi:10.1111/j.1525-139X.2007.00349.x. PMID 17991192.

Sharifi-Mollayousefi A, Yazdchi-Marandi M, Ayramlou H, et al. (February 2008). "Assessment of body mass index and hand anthropometric measurements as independent risk factors for carpal tunnel syndrome". Folia Morphol. (Warsz) 67 (1): 36–42. PMID 18335412.

Shaw K, Gennat H, O'Rourke P, Del Mar C (2006). "Exercise for overweight or obesity". Cochrane database of systematic reviews (Online) (4): CD003817. doi:10.1002/14651858.CD003817.pub3. PMID 17054187.

Shick SM, Wing RR, Klem ML, McGuire MT, Hill JO, Seagle H (April 1998). "Persons successful at long-term weight loss and maintenance continue to consume a low-energy, low-fat diet". J Am Diet Assoc 98 (4): 408–13. doi:10.1016/S0002-8223(98)00093-5. PMID 9550162.

Shoelson SE, Herrero L, Naaz A (May 2007). "Obesity, inflammation, and insulin resistance". Gastroenterology 132 (6): 2169–80. doi:10.1053/j.gastro.2007.03.059. PMID 17498510.

Shoelson SE, Lee J, Goldfine AB (July 2006). "Inflammation and insulin resistance". J. Clin. Invest. 116 (7): 1793–801. doi:10.1172/JCI29069. PMID 16823477. PMC 1483173. http://www.jci.org/articles/view/29069.

Sjöström L, Narbro K, Sjöström CD, et al. (2007). "Effects of bariatric surgery on mortality in Swedish obese subjects". N. Engl. J. Med. 357 (8): 741–52. doi:10.1056/NEJMoa066254. PMID 17715408.

Sjöström L, Narbro K, Sjöström CD, et al. (August 2007). "Effects of bariatric surgery on mortality in Swedish obese subjects". N. Engl. J. Med. 357 (8): 741–52. doi:10.1056/NEJMoa066254. PMID 17715408.

Snow V, Barry P, Fitterman N, Qaseem A, Weiss K (2005). "Pharmacologic and surgical management of obesity in primary care: A clinical practice guideline from the American College of Physicians". Ann Intern Med 142 (7): 525–31. PMID 15809464. Fulltext.

Sobal J, Stunkard AJ (March 1989). "Socioeconomic status and obesity: A review of the literature". Psychol Bull 105 (2): 260–75. doi:10.1037/0033-2909.105.2.260. PMID 2648443.

Strychar I (January 2006). "Diet in the management of weight loss". CMAJ 174 (1): 56–63. doi:10.1503/cmaj.045037. PMID 16389240. PMC 1319349. http://www.cmaj.ca/cgi/content/full/174/1/56.

Sturm R (July 2007). "Increases in morbid obesity in the USA: 2000–2005". Public Health 121 (7): 492–6. doi:10.1016/j.puhe.2007.01.006. PMID 17399752.

Sweeting HN (2007). "Measurement and definitions of obesity in childhood and adolescence: A field guide for the uninitiated". Nutr J 6: 32. doi:10.1186/1475-2891-6-32. PMID 17963490. PMC 2164947. http://www.nutritionj.com/content/6/1/32.

Tate DF, Jeffery RW, Sherwood NE, Wing RR (1 April 2007). "Long-term weight losses associated with prescription of higher physical activity goals. Are higher levels of physical activity protective against weight regain?". Am. J. Clin. Nutr. 85 (4): 954–9. PMID 17413092. http://www.ajcn.org/cgi/content/full/85/4/954.

Theodore Mazzone; Giamila Fantuzzi (2006). Adipose Tissue And Adipokines in Health And Disease (Nutrition and Health). Totowa, NJ: Humana Press. pp. 222. ISBN 1-58829-721-7.

Tice JA, Karliner L, Walsh J, Petersen AJ, Feldman MD (October 2008). "Gastric banding or bypass? A systematic review comparing the two most popular bariatric procedures". Am. J. Med. 121 (10): 885–93. doi:10.1016/j.amjmed.2008.05.036. PMID 18823860.

Tjepkema M (2005-07-06). "Measured Obesity–Adult obesity in Canada: Measured height and weight". Nutrition: Findings from the Canadian Community Health Survey. Ottawa, Ontario: Statistics Canada. http://www.statcan.gc.ca/pub/82-620-m/2005001/article/adults-adultes/8060-eng.htm.

Tsai AG, Wadden TA (January 2005). "Systematic review: an evaluation of major commercial weight loss programs in the United States". Ann. Intern. Med. 142 (1): 56–66. PMID 15630109.

Tsigosa Constantine; Hainer, Vojtech; Basdevant, Arnaud; Finer, Nick; Fried, Martin; Mathus-Vliegen, Elisabeth; Micic, Dragan; Maislos, Maximo et al. (April 2008). "Management of Obesity in Adults: European Clinical Practice Guidelines". The European Journal of Obesity 1: 106. doi:10.1159/000126822.

Tucker LA, Bagwell M (July 1991). "Television viewing and obesity in adult females" (PDF). Am J Public Health 81 (7): 908–11. doi:10.2105/AJPH.81.7.908. PMID 2053671. PMC 1405200. http://www.ajph.org/cgi/reprint/81/7/908.

Tukker A, Visscher T, Picavet H (April 2008). "Overweight and health problems of the lower extremities: osteoarthritis, pain and disability". Public Health Nutr 12 (3): 1–10. doi:10.1017/S1368980008002103. PMID 18426630.

U.S. Preventive Services Task Force (June 2003). "Behavioral counseling in primary care to promote a healthy diet: recommendations and rationale" ([dead link]). Am Fam Physician 67 (12): 2573–6. PMID 12825847. http://www.aafp.org/afp/20030615/us.html.

UK Prospective Diabetes Study (UKPDS) Group (1998). "Effect of intensive blood-glucose control with metformin on complications in overweight patients with type 2 diabetes (UKPDS 34)". Lancet 352 (9131): 854–65. doi:10.1016/S0140-6736(98)07037-8. PMID 9742977.

Van Baal PH, Polder JJ, de Wit GA, et al. (February 2008). "Lifetime medical costs of obesity: Prevention no cure for increasing health expenditure". PLoS Med. 5 (2): e29.

doi:10.1371/journal.pmed.0050029. PMID 18254654. PMC 2225430.
http://www.plosmedicine.org/article/info:doi/10.1371/journal.pmed.0050029.

Vioque J, Torres A, Quiles J (December 2000). "Time spent watching television, sleep duration and obesity in adults living in Valencia, Spain". Int. J. Obes. Relat. Metab. Disord. 24 (12): 1683–8. doi:10.1038/sj.ijo.0801434. PMID 11126224.

Wall M (March 2008). "Idiopathic intracranial hypertension (pseudotumor cerebri)". Curr Neurol Neurosci Rep 8 (2): 87–93. doi:10.1007/s11910-008-0015-0. PMID 18460275.

Walley AJ, Asher JE, Froguel P (June 2009). "The genetic contribution to non-syndromic human obesity". Nat. Rev. Genet. 10 (7): 431–42. doi:10.1038/nrg2594. PMID 19506576.

Wanless, Sir Derek; John Appleby, Anthony Harrison, Darshan Patel (2007). Our Future Health Secured? A review of NHS funding and performance. London, UK: The King's Fund. ISBN 185717562X. http://www.kingsfund.org.uk/research/publications/our_future.html. Retrieved 2007-12-17.

Weiss EC, Galuska DA, Kettel Khan L, Gillespie C, Serdula MK (July 2007). "Weight regain in U.S. adults who experienced substantial weight loss, 1999–2002". Am J Prev Med 33 (1): 34–40. doi:10.1016/j.amepre.2007.02.040. PMID 17572309.

Wells JC (February 2009). "Ethnic variability in adiposity and cardiovascular risk: the variable disease selection hypothesis". Int J Epidemiol 38 (1): 63–71. doi:10.1093/ije/dyn183. PMID 18820320.

Weng HH, Bastian LA, Taylor DH, Moser BK, Ostbye T (2004). "Number of children associated with obesity in middle-aged women and men: results from the health and retirement study". J Womens Health (Larchmt) 13 (1): 85–91. doi:10.1089/154099904322836492. PMID 15006281.

Whitlock G, Lewington S, Sherliker P, et al. (March 2009). "Body-mass index and cause-specific mortality in 900 000 adults: collaborative analyses of 57 prospective studies". Lancet 373 (9669): 1083–96. doi:10.1016/S0140-6736(09)60318-4. PMID 19299006.

Wilkinson, Richard; Pickett, Kate (2009). The Spirit Level: Why More Equal Societies Almost Always Do Better. London: Allen Lane. pp. 91–101. ISBN 978-1-846-14039-6. http://www.equalitytrust.org.uk/why/evidence/obesity.

Williamson DF, Pamuk E, Thun M, Flanders D, Byers T, Heath C (June 1995). "Prospective study of intentional weight loss and mortality in never-smoking overweight US white women aged 40–64 years". Am. J. Epidemiol. 141 (12): 1128–41. PMID 7771451.

Wing, Rena R; Phelan, Suzanne (1 July 2005). "Science-Based Solutions to Obesity: What are the Roles of Academia, Government, Industry, and Health Care? Proceedings of a symposium, Boston, Massachusetts, USA, 10–11 March 2004 and Anaheim, California, USA, 2 October 2004". Am. J. Clin. Nutr. 82 (1 Suppl): 207S–273S. PMID 16002825. http://www.ajcn.org/cgi/content/full/82/1/222S.

Woodhouse R (2008). "Obesity in art: A brief overview". Front Horm Res 36: 271–86. doi:10.1159/000115370. PMID 18230908. http://books.google.ca/books?id=nXRU4Ea1aMkC&pg=PA271&lpg=PA271&dq=Obesity+in+a rt:+a+brief+overview&source=web&ots=G2ofZTj__r&sig=7HbW8aAnoQ-RIwt09ocD3xOHJZU&hl=en&sa=X&oi=book_result&resnum=5&ct=result#PPA271,M1.

Wright JD, Kennedy-Stephenson J, Wang CY, McDowell MA, Johnson CL (February 2004). "Trends in intake of energy and macronutrients—United States, 1971–2000". MMWR Morb Mortal Wkly Rep 53 (4): 80–2. PMID 14762332. http://www.cdc.gov/mmwr/preview/mmwrhtml/mm5304a3.htm.

Yach D, Stuckler D, Brownell KD (January 2006). "Epidemiologic and economic consequences of the global epidemics of obesity and diabetes". Nat. Med. 12 (1): 62–6. doi:10.1038/nm0106-62. PMID 16397571.

Yang W, Kelly T, He J (2007). "Genetic epidemiology of obesity". Epidemiol Rev 29: 49–61. doi:10.1093/epirev/mxm004. PMID 17566051.

Yosipovitch G, DeVore A, Dawn A (June 2007). "Obesity and the skin: skin physiology and skin manifestations of obesity". J. Am. Acad. Dermatol. 56 (6): 901–16; quiz 917–20. doi:10.1016/j.jaad.2006.12.004. PMID 17504714.

Yusuf S, Hawken S, Ounpuu S, Dans T, Avezum A, Lanas F, McQueen M, Budaj A, Pais P, Varigos J, Lisheng L, INTERHEART Study Investigators. (2004). "Effect of potentially modifiable risk factors associated with myocardial infarction in 52 countries (the INTERHEART study): Case-control study". Lancet 364 (9438): 937–52. doi:10.1016/S0140-6736(04)17018-9. PMID 15364185.

Zachary Bloomgarden (2003). "Prevention of Obesity and Diabetes". Diabetes Care 26 (11): 3172–3178. doi:10.2337/diacare.26.11.3172. PMID 14578257. http://care.diabetesjournals.org/content/26/11/3172.full.

Zametkin AJ, Zoon CK, Klein HW, Munson S (February 2004). "Psychiatric aspects of child and adolescent obesity: a review of the past 10 years". J Am Acad Child Adolesc Psychiatry 43 (2): 134–50. doi:10.1097/01.chi.0000100427.25002.06 (inactive 2009-04-10). PMID 14726719.

Disclaimer

The content of this book is intended for educational and information purposes only. As such, any of the information contained herein should not be accepted as a substitute for the advice of qualified physicians in the treatment and management of obesity and any related conditions.

References in this book to names of celebrities, either living or deceased, with respect to the subject of obesity were derived from information that is considered public domain. Such references were offered merely as case points and, in no instance were intended to offend or to specifically exemplify these individuals as this relates to their condition.

The content of this book was derived from prevailing research and scientific knowledge; however, any inaccuracies or exceptions of fact which may be perceived from the manner in which such information is conveyed or presented was not, in any way, intended by the author.

Index

About the Author

Dorothy S. "Carol" Mukherjee considers herself an ordinary person, but her passion for health and wellness is quite extraordinary as the content of this book should demonstrate. Born in Charlotte, North Carolina, Dorothy Mukherjee is the second of five children, including two brothers and two sisters. Her propensity for helping others led her to Watts School of Nursing from which she earned the distinction as a registered nurse. After working for a while as a surgical nurse, Carol moved on to manage a dialysis center in Kissimmee, Florida. Meanwhile she completed her Bachelor of Arts degree in Psychology. Her interest in obesity derived primarily from the struggles of her father and mother who both died from complications related to obesity, including diabetes and cancer. Struggling with similar challenges in her own life, Carol devoted years to studying obesity, its causes and its consequences. She is a staunch advocate and supporter of wellness and preventive-health programs for persons struggling with obesity and has dedicated this book to their plight.

OBESITY

It Might Not Be ALL Your Fault,
But It IS Your Problem …

For everything you've ever wanted to know about obesity, this is it. Presented in an easy-to-read, user-friendly writing style, this book takes a comprehensive look at the problem of obesity. It progressively invites the reader into a detailed explanation of obesity, including how it is measured, its causes, its complications and how it can lead to other serious medical problems. The book also addresses the historical, cultural and social aspects of obesity and how its prevalence in modern times is influenced by industry, urbanism, population, media and even social interaction. Finally, the book addresses the many alternative approaches to managing and curing obesity, including a logical procedure for losing and sustaining one's desired weight. As a bonus, the book includes a detailed food calorie chart as well as an activity chart by which one can determine how many calories are burned through various types of physical activity.

Not only is this an excellent source of educational content, but also a handy library reference for anyone who struggles with the problem of obesity, for doctors, nurses and therapists who manage obesity and even for those who just want to learn about the magnitude of the problem.